Oh Behave!

Dogs from Pavlov to Premack to Pinker

Jean Donaldson

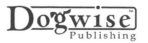
Publishing

Wenatchee, WA

Oh Behave! Dogs from Pavlov to Premack to Pinker
Jean Donaldson

Dogwise Publishing
A Division of Direct Book Service, Inc.
701B Poplar Wenatchee, Washington 98801
1-509-663-9115, 1-800-776-2665
www.dogwisepublishing.com / info@dogwisepublishing.com
© 2008 Jean Donaldson

Graphic Design: Nathan Woodward & Lindsay Peternell
Cover Design and Photo: Craig McMahon
Illustrations: Verne K. Foster
Index: Cheryl Smith

Limits of Liability and Disclaimer of Warranty:
The author and publisher shall not be liable in the event of incidental or consequential damages in connection with, or arising out of, the furnishing, performance, or use of the instructions and suggestions contained in this book.

Library of Congress Cataloging-in-Publication Data

Donaldson, Jean.
Oh behave! : dogs from Pavlov to Premack to Pinker / Jean Donaldson.
p. cm.
Includes bibliographical references and index.
ISBN 978-1-929242-52-8 (alk. paper)
1. Dogs--Behavior. 2. Dogs--Psychology. 3. Dogs--Training. I. Title.
SF433.D68 2008
636.7'089689--dc22
2008006637

ISBN10: 1-929242-52-2
ISBN13: 978-1-929242-52-8

Printed in the U.S.A.

Author's Note

This book began as an intersection of the two great loves of my life: dogs and evolution. For years I rolled around in my head how to convey how exciting and omni-relevant I find evolution to people who are, like me, avid students of dogs and behavior. In a small way, this is the result of that effort.

The other piece of the book is my attempt, where I am able, to dig up answers to questions I hear or am sent about dog training and behavior. Identifying features of such cases have been altered to protect anonymity while I tried to preserve the essence of the question, what that person was really wanting to know. There is also a bit of editorializing, which, although potentially irksome to readers who do not share my biases, I hope are thoughtful stabs at some of the issues in the dog training field. I in no way am under the illusion that I have any monopoly on truth.

Jean Donaldson
December 19, 2007

Table of Contents

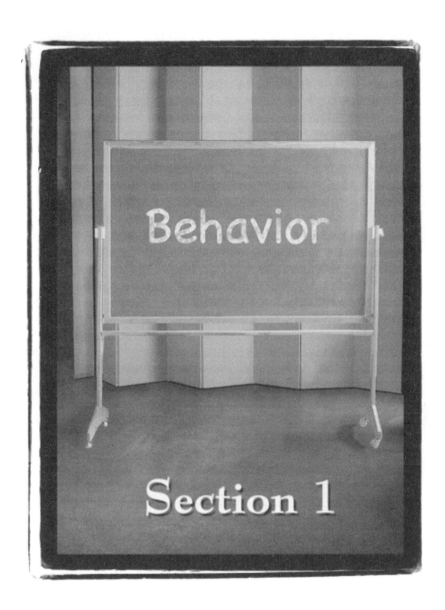

Behavior

Section 1

Chemistry and Constraints: How We Choose Our Dogs

A student film-maker came to the San Francisco SPCA the other day to shoot a documentary on Pit Bulls. She interviewed a staff member, Christine, who had a six-year old Pit named Bug. The film-maker asked her how she came to choose Bug. Christine replied, "Oh, I grew up with Pit Bulls." All of us looking on nodded sagely, as though that was a clear explanation.

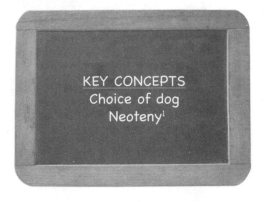

KEY CONCEPTS
Choice of dog
Neoteny[1]

Then I got to thinking. I grew up with creamed corn, cats, budgies, and a Doberman. None of these has made a recent appearance in my house. It can't simply be only about what one has gotten used to. So, what does determine our dog choices?

There's a substantial body of research on mate selection in everything from fruit flies to mice to quail to humans, however I'm not sure we can glean much about dog selection from this. So, using a wholly unrigorous approach—mulling it over in the shower and chatting with some dog friends—I have generated the following list of dog choice factors.

[1]Neoteny is the retention into adulthood of juvenile or infantile traits—they can be "morphological" (body shape, also known as pedomorphosis) traits such as floppy ears and the facial features of the breeds mentioned, or behavioral, such as barking and the tendency to lick faces.

Factor 1: What Floats Your Boat

Ah, Chemistry. I have vivid memories of pressing my face to a pet store window as a child, longing for the miniature longhaired Dachshund puppy behind the glass. As an adult I would never patronize a pet store that sells dogs, however mini longhaired Dachsies still make me weak in the knees. I've also been known to scream when a really nice Peke enters the conformation ring. The ideal specimen for me has the appearance of being from another planet. "Eeeeeeee!!!! I must have one! I must have one!" I can also get all soft-focus for a well-groomed Maltese or a Toy Poodle that in any way resembles a lamb.

A friend of mine loves all things Rottie. Even individuals that wildly diverge from the breed standard, not to mention from what most people would think of as a handsome dog, make her giddy. Undershot, crazy leggy, it doesn't matter. Not surprisingly, she has rescued a couple of hard-luck Rotties and Rottie-like dogs in the time I've known her. Another friend of mine digs Boston Terriers and French Bulldogs. The key criterion in her case seems to be the neotenous (squishy puppy-like) facial features. For this very reason she has squealed next to me while at ringside during Pekes.

Chemistry seems to come first and then may be followed by a seamless narrative of logical-sounding rationalizations, preserving the illusion that we decided to adopt a litter of Jack Russell Terriers for quite excellent reasons. This effect wreaks havoc for animal shelter staff who must play bad cop when aisle-shoppers fall for a face owned by a dog that is completely inappropriate for their life situation.

Factor 2: Constraints

As a child I begged, lobbied, and extorted in my attempts to secure a dog, preferably a Papillon, mini Dachsie, or variation on the lamb theme, but was disallowed by my parents. Then my father visited a relative in Calgary who happened to be into Dobies. Clearly the dogs in the house won him over because he returned home to declare that I could have a Doberman. Okay, so it was not a miniature Dachshund. But it had a leg on each corner, a tail (sort of) and I could actually have one. Done.

Family members, including resident dogs, usually have veto power, which can significantly narrow the field. Spouses, for instance, are very often in the role of Constrainer of Breed. I swoon for Chinese Cresteds but, alas, I'm not allowed by my husband. A woman I know in Virginia experienced, as an adult, a variation on my childhood theme, played out with her husband who didn't want any dog in the house until he became besotted with Cavalier King Charles Spaniels. Didn't have to ask her twice. She had a Cavalier within minutes. And we all know people whose spouses impose a number cap. Which is not necessarily a bad thing.

Factor 3: Love the One You're With

I've long observed a funny thing about groups of people. Put them together and they inevitably make friends with each other and start pairing up as mates. It is a rare person who, like a cast member of "Lost," doesn't end up with any friends or lovers from the pool of people they're in regular contact with. Very much blows apart the one soul-mate-in-the-universe theory.

This is to my mind the explanation for Extremely Long Term Foster Phenomenon, i.e., the Chow is Staying. Had you asked me, prior to getting Buffy, my Chow, if I would ever, in a million years, under any circumstances, have a Chow, the answer would have been no. Unequivocal no. In fact, when colleagues chided me about fostering a puppy and getting all bonded and keeping her, I laughed and laughed at their naiveté. I'd fostered and had in my home for training scores of dogs and only a small handful were ever difficult to give back. I got to know them all and loved them, all but keep them? Ha ha ha ha ha!!! My laughter rang in the corridor as I toted off the carrier with my ferocious little charge inside. "No risk here—it's a Chow!"

Fast forward five years. I'm all about Chows. Never say never.

Factor 4: Readiness

My friend Janis had flirted with the idea of adopting a retired racing Greyhound for a couple of years before the time was right for her. When she was down to one dog—a Def Con II situation— and had finished the project she vowed to complete before going dog shopping, she was ready. A couple of rescue groups had dogs available. The second or third dog she met got along with the resident dog (constraint) and was snapped up. Lucky dog. We should all want to be reincarnated as one of Janis's dogs.

After the loss of a dog, people vary enormously in their readiness to bring home someone new. I know people who've taken years to feel ready and others who can't bear—not for a day—to be without a dog, so are combing sources literally within hours of losing a cherished pet. I've often thought that people who feel as though their dogs chose them, or that fate intervened when a dog dropped into their lives, might have been ready, but didn't know it until a dog came along. One day the perfect storm of factors may converge and I'll have my miniature longhaired Dachshund. Heart be still.

Test Your Dog's IQ

Although I never tire of quoting one of my heroes, cognitive neuroscientist Steven Pinker, that intelligence is but one act in nature's talent show (ours), like most dog people, I notice what I think are differences in cleverness between dogs. So, for fun, I checked out various dog IQ tests, reviewed the dog cognition research and,

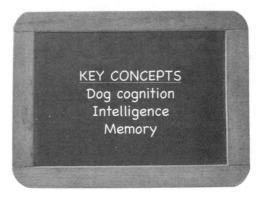

KEY CONCEPTS
Dog cognition
Intelligence
Memory

drawing ideas from both, created the following. Disclaimer: this is strictly for fun. Whereas human SAT tests predict grade point average in your freshman year of college, what follows has not been shown to predict anything at all.

Problem Solving One—Paws or No?

You will need a timer and a legged sofa or chair with a gap at the bottom low enough that your dog cannot fit his head into but, if he tried, could reach into with his paws. The idea is to see if he will indeed attempt the latter to get at something underneath.

Show your dog a tasty treat or a new toy, and make sure he sees you put it under the sofa, far enough that he can't bite it, but close enough for him to touch it with his paws.

Now egg him on to get it. If he does nothing at all, he scores zero. If he tries with his mouth without any twisting of his head or body and then gives up, give him a one. If he tries more variations on the mouth theme, notably twisting his head to different degrees to make it fit, but never moves on to paws, score it a two. If he uses his paws to reach under but fails to get the item, give him a three. If he gets the item with his paws in thirty or more seconds, give him a four. If he gets the item with his paws in less than thirty seconds, he gets a five.

Wait twenty-four hours and then run the test again. Does he improve on his previous strategy? If yes, give him a bonus point.

Problem Solving Two—Fence Test

This item will test whether your dog can employ a detour. You'll need a novel fence that he can see through and that is at least forty feet long (the detour therefore being twenty feet to either side from the center). With you centered on the other side, call him to you and time how long it takes him—if ever—to make the sideways detour. It's better if he doesn't observe you taking the detour to your station. A toy or food throw perpendicular to the center of the fence will temporarily distract him so you can get yourself placed.

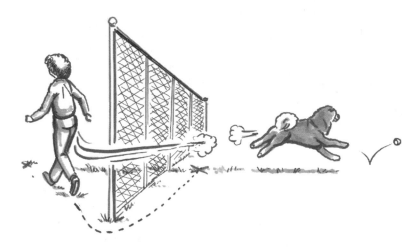

Once he arrives at the fence and sees you on the other side, start the timer. If he hasn't gone around after a minute, coach him: take a few steps in one direction and gesture.

Score him a zero if he doesn't take the detour even with the prompting at the one minute mark. Score him a one if he succeeds but required prompting. Score two if he does it on his own between the thirty-second and one-minute marks, a three if he does it within thirty seconds and a four if he takes the detour right away. Add one point to any score if he has never, ever done any fence detour such as this before.

Repeat the test twenty-four hours later and give him a bonus point if he upgrades his performance.

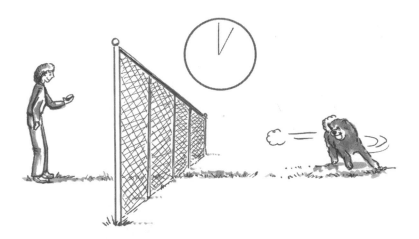

Memory Test—Where's the Goodie?

This will test how long your dog can remember a specific spot. To prep, play a game where you let him watch you hide a cookie and then let him get it. For instance, jam a cookie between two sofa cushions and then let him nose it out and eat it. Repeat this in a number of places, ones that he wouldn't normally investigate and that, if he hadn't seen you place the cookie, wouldn't know it was there without sniffing. Once he's learned that he can take these cookies, start the test.

Put a cookie in a new place, letting him see you do it as usual, but right after doing so, take him out of the house for one minute. As soon as a minute has passed, let him back in and see if he beelines for the cookie. It doesn't count as "beelining" if he sniffs it out later. He has to go directly to the spot. Using a new hiding place each time, repeat with a two-minute, three-minute, four-minute, and then one-hour lag. If he doesn't get any of the cookies, give him zero. If he gets the one-minute cookie, he scores a one, the two-minute cookie a two, the three-minute a three, and the four-minute a four. If he remembers where the cookie is after one hour on errands, give him a five.

Inference Test

An inference is a deduction that is formed without direct evidence. It is a talent all normal humans have in spades. To test whether your dog can perform a rudimentary inference you will need soft, tasty treats and two bowls, placed three or four feet apart. Put your dog on a stay, or tether him so he is ten feet from the bowl set-up. Smear both bowls with some treat, so they both smell. With him watching, make a big show of putting a treat under one of the bowls. Then, station yourself in the middle between the bowls, release him from the stay (or go un-tether him) and watch closely. Does he beeline to the correct bowl? If yes, lift the bowl and let him get the treat. If he goes to the wrong bowl, lift it so he discovers there is nothing there, then wait until he investigates the correct bowl. When he does, lift it so he can have the treat. Repeat this ten times, randomly alternating which bowl the treat is under, and keep track of what he does each time. Now, do another ten repetitions, but this time, don't let him see you place the treat (be sneaky). What you will let him see before releasing him is a big show of you lifting up the other bowl, the one without the treat. Then release him. Does he go to the bowl you were fussing with (the bowl without the treat) or to the treat bowl? Repeat this game ten times and keep score.

He scores zero if his overall performance on the twenty trials is no better than chance (i.e. with pure guesswork he'd be right half the time). Score him a one if he is initially not very good at the first exercise, but improves over the ten repetitions, and performs in reverse (usually going for the wrong bowl) on the second exercise.

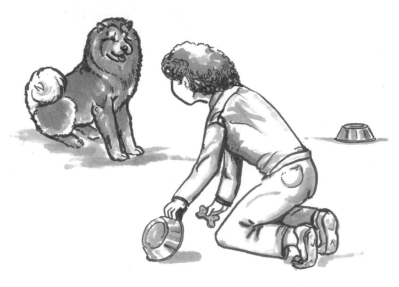

Score him a two if he improves during the first exercise and then starts performing in reverse on the second exercise, but improves (to chance or better) over the ten repetitions. Score him a three if he nails the first exercise (ten for ten), but performs in reverse on the second. He gets a four if his first exercise is perfect and he improves over the course of the second and a five if he nails both exercises.

Results

16 to 20	Crazy clever
10 to 15	Clever
6 to 9	Normal
0 to 5	Getting by on looks

Observation vs. Interpretation

Dear Jean,

Sydney is an eight month old American Cocker. He loves jumping on the bed and walking on my husband and me in the morning. He never jumps on the bed when we're not in it. My class instructor says he thinks he is establishing his dominance and that we should disallow it, crate him over-

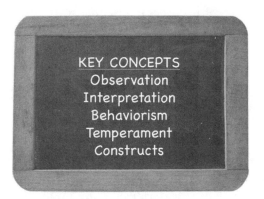

KEY CONCEPTS
Observation
Interpretation
Behaviorism
Temperament
Constructs

night, and show more leadership. My husband says he's pretending to be hunting for birds. I used to think he was just having fun, but I now wonder if Sydney has realized that this is a good way to get our attention. What is he thinking?

I don't know. I can't know. I, you, your husband, your trainer, and the top fifty dog gurus on the planet cannot know what Sydney is thinking. This is not a dodge. In fact, not only is it not a dodge, it's a concession that is made far too seldom in dog behavior circles.

What Sydney is doing—"jumping on the bed when people are in it and walking on the people"—is an observation. We can all witness it, quantify it (how many steps, for how long, at what time of day, etc.); and agree that that is what he is doing. In contrast to observations are interpretations, which are attempted explanations about why he is doing what he is doing. Interpretations are stabs at the dog's internal events—emotions and thoughts that mediate behavior. These internal events cannot be observed, even with access to brain scanning technology, which can only record correlates (like blood flow in specific regions) to other observable events (like behavior or a person's stated thoughts). In the domestic dog behavior community, there is a veritable cottage industry in interpreting what dogs do. The part that concerns me is the way many of these guesses are passed off as fact or strongly supported theory.

No one can "observe" that a dog is establishing dominance or pretending to hunt for birds, thinking a particular thought, or even that the dog is thinking at all (including in pictures). These are all interpretations. One can observe that a dog is jumping on a bed and walking around under certain circumstances. One can observe facial expressions, vocalizations, and differences in the environment that make him more or less likely to do it or stop doing it. One can then generate hypotheses about why he does it. Interpretations are kind of like hypotheses that never undergo testing the way formal hypotheses do.

Interpretations are useful insofar as they help us "chunk" observations into useful constructs—rather than saying "the dog put his front legs parallel to the ground, opened his mouth on the horizontal axis by two and one half inches past baseline, held his tail at ten degrees past vertical and moved it at a frequency of six cycles per second and an amplitude of…" we say "the dog is soliciting play." This is an interpretation, in this case one that is well supported by replicable observation of what happens next when virtually all dogs do this behavior.

This chunking in turn helps us to understand behavior in a deeper, more meaningful way. The danger with interpretations of hidden events—especially of the "one dog did this once" variety—is that they are notoriously difficult to falsify. No one can prove you wrong. The philosopher Bertrand Russell once mused that there was a small china teapot in perfect elliptical orbit around the sun. No one can prove him wrong so it might very well be there. The question then becomes, "is it likely?" The maxim in science is "big claims need big evidence."

There is some merit to sticking to observations as much as possible and avoiding the temptation to invent interpretations, however intuitive they might feel. This tendency to stick to observations for pragmatic purposes is known as behaviorism. Behaviorism put forward the idea of a black box—the animal's internal machinations— and that understanding of these inner workings were not necessary in order to conceptualize and, ultimately, control behavior. It's not true that behaviorists deny there is anything going on in the black box of the animal's brain. It's that they don't think it's necessary or particularly relevant when it comes to modifying behavior. Behaviorism has fallen wildly out of favor in psychology, but is extremely useful in one particular domain of relevance to us doggie people: animal training.

Opinions, not surprisingly, differ when it comes to interpreting dog behavior. One fantastic example is dogs that growl, snarl, or snap when approached while eating or chewing a bone. An interpreter from the behaviorism school would say "the dog growled when the approacher came within five feet and from the dog's right." Another interpreter would say "the dog is displaying his dominance." The latter would likely lay out a plan to lower the dog's presumed status in the family hierarchy, whereas the behaviorist would lay out a modification strategy to stop the dog growling when he's approached with a bone.

Another example comes from the animal sheltering world. The prevailing culture is one of ascribing character traits rather than describing what dogs do while in the shelter or during an intake test. The very terms used to describe tests that shelters use belie their bias for or against behaviorism. For instance, being of the behaviorist ilk, at the San Francisco SPCA we conduct "Behavior Evaluations," which are quantified tests of what dogs do when, for example, approached while eating, handled on various parts of their body, or when meeting another dog. Many other shelters conduct "Temperament Tests," which may use similar scenarios, but frame testee responses more in terms of set, unyielding traits the dog has rather than something the dog did. Dogs are "dominant," "submissive," "pushy," etc. rather than doing X, Y, or Z.

Supporters of the fixed temperament construct feel they have un-
covered a dog's immutable essence with the right test, whereas behaviorists are more inclined to think that "this is what the dog did
in this circumstance on this day." They will then measure whether
this is predictive of behavior in the adopter's home. Behaviorists
are also more likely to then ask, "do you want more or less of this
behavior" and proceed to change it. Fixed temperament aficionados
might feel that a dog who performs well on a temperament test
after training or behavior modification has (presumably danger-
ously) had his true nature masked whereas a behaviorist would, on
the same basis, question the value of the "temperament" construct
in this context.

Regardless of who is right, there is no denying that humans are
drawn to the idea of "temperament." Humans got in line twice for
doses of what psychologists call "theory of mind"—the ability to
imagine the internal events of someone else, and we seem to project
madly and gleefully across species lines. Discussions about temperament, for instance, are far from unique to dogs. Hamster people
don't just describe what hamsters do, they refer to different hamster
temperaments, as do hobbyists who are into gerbils, hedgehogs,
snakes, salamanders, box turtles, guppies, goldfish, and iguanas
("iguanas that are switched from small cages to free-roaming demonstrate an improvement in temperament"). Even tarantula owners
describe their charges as "secretive," "cautious," "methodical,"
"peaceful," and "spunky" rather than observing and quantifying
tarantula behavior. Box turtles are described as "full of personality."
Goldfish, too, have "loads of personality" and one even, according
to the owner "discovered that bubbles are fun."

Interpreting behavior, quite aside from its usefulness, is so reinforcing to people it is unlikely to diminish any time soon. There are,
however, small signs of increasing circumspection about the guesses
dog people make about dog behavior, which is no doubt very reinforcing to behaviorists. The bottom line is for all of us to know the
difference between observations and interpretations and to be up
front about labeling interpretations as such when we make them.

Wolf Behavior Patterns— Some Dogs Got 'Em, Some Dogs Not So Much

Dear Jean,

My Shiba Inu, Jordan, "buries" certain of his toys in the sofa cushion. I use quotations because at the end of several minutes of labor the toy is often still clearly visible. But that never stops him from doing it again and again, always pushing imaginary dirt over it after carefully inserting it

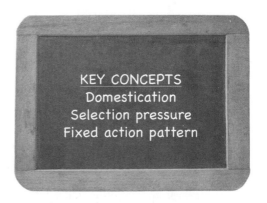

KEY CONCEPTS
Domestication
Selection pressure
Fixed action pattern

in his chosen spot. Then, sometimes after doing all this to some chew object, he'll take it out and chew on it right away, rendering all his effort a waste. This is the first dog I've had that buries anything. He's no more into his toys than the others were. Why does he do it when the others didn't?

Fabulously interesting! An even better question would be: why don't all dogs cache food? Or guard it from rivals, including us? Or howl? Why only some?

The reason is domestication. Whereas humans have exerted formidable selection pressure on dogs vis-a-vis their body shapes, sizes, coat features, and certain precisely defined utilitarian behaviors, other pressures, such as for traits that would help a dog make a living in a wild environment, have been relaxed. Put it this way: virtually 100% of red foxes have a nice, strong, highly stereotyped food-caching behavior. They will bury unused food portions using a standardized set of actions and then return to them later. This standardized set of actions common to all members of a species is called a fixed action pattern (FAP). Fixed action patterns require no learning though sometimes will become refined with practice. Eminently useful, like bundled software. Foxcs born with mutations that weaken or edit out FAPs, like food-caching, are at a sufficient disadvantage in that they tend to not live long enough to pass on this variation to their offspring. So the gene(s) for the trait fixes at 100% frequency in the population. In dogs, by contrast, any such mutation would be invisible to evolution, i.e., neutral: dogs like Jordan, who retain the trait from food-caching wolf ancestors, provided they passed muster with regards to designated breeding criteria, would pass it on, and—this is important—so would dogs without the burying tendency. Think of it as a social safety net for non-food-caching dogs.

This same effect can result in a partially retained or inexpertly targeted fixed action pattern, such as Jordan's rather feckless choice of sofa and air as media, and his immediate consumption (never mind that many dogs do it, as Jordon does, with non-food items, inefficient at best in cost-benefit terms). Dogs are treasure troves of behaviors that have drifted all over the map in the absence of certain key selection pressures. The predatory behavior department also abounds with great examples. While selection pressure has been exerted in certain breeds to magnify pieces of the wolf predation sequence—think herding, pointing, retrieving, and terriers grimly hanging on—others have been left to drift. Most dogs no longer hunt for a living. And so some dogs, like Border Collies, are turned on by any moving object, some by moving critters only, and some by nothing. Many dogs will perform a grab-and-shake on a toy, a nifty neck-breaking behavior for small prey items, but not all dogs do. It's a safe bet that 100% of wolves have more than a passing interest in critters, and can dispatch small prey.

Carcass dissection appears in a percentage of dogs, usually in the form of evisceration of stuffed animals. Many of us have had dogs that, once given a stuffy, expertly render it into scores of bits within fifteen minutes. And many of us have also had dogs that, ten years later, still tote around the same Mr. Squirrelly. Clearly missing the dissection chip. Some dogs relish a good roll on a carcass or in manure and others, happily, not so much.

Reproductive behavior is another realm of some interesting diversity in dogs. Not all dogs can successfully reproduce unassisted. While in many such cases this is a collateral effect of unhelpful conformation, in others the barrier is behavioral rather than anatomical. One interesting example is a range of perseverance in males. Due to the nature of the estrous cycle in dogs, bitches are highly attractive before they are receptive. Ian Dunbar has proposed that this early-in-cycle onset of attractiveness is an adaptation in free-ranging dogs to accumulate suitors and then vet them for fitness. It's in her genetic interest to have some significant choice of fathers when she's finally receptive, and as free-ranging dogs appear to be fairly nomadic, this may take some time. A possible result of this is the evolution in such populations of a stronger than average if-at-first-you-don't-succeed-try-again trait in males: if they're snarked (trainer-speak for a snarl-bark hybrid) off once, do they take their marbles and go home or do they bounce back and persevere ("How about now??). Those in the latter group will still be present when she finally becomes receptive. Enter selective breeding. If he's handsome and clever to humans, it matters not that he is a total giver-upper: we'll get him bred to her somehow.

Maternal coprophagia—the consumption by a dam of neonate elimination products—has been retained in many dogs, as has the co-evolved trait in neonate puppies of being unable to eliminate without licking stimulation by their dam. The fitness significance of this behavior is likely two-fold: lowering of disease risk through better hygiene and better predator avoidance due to the waste-free nest's lower olfactory profile.

In contrast to widely retained maternal coprophagia is regurgitation. 100% of adult wolves in a pack, including aunts and uncles, will regurgitate food if puppies paw and lick at their mouths when they return from hunting. This behavior is only occasionally seen in nursing bitches and, even more rarely, in other adult dogs. It's possible that this trait drifted more than maternal coprophagia because of greater across-the-board sustenance support in early human-reared dog populations, i.e., the safety net of food was more steadily supplied than house-cleaning services. The pressure remained on the latter trait and forced its retention.

And, speaking of starvation, the tendency to gorge, i.e., eat waaaaay more than required for immediate energy needs, has clearly been retained in dogs judging by the epidemic of obesity in our pets. Wolves are subject to a feast-famine lifestyle where it is highly adaptive to tank up when food is available, but remove the famine part, as with pet dogs, and the pounds pile on. Our human fondness for foods high in fat and sugar is similarly a retained and now maladaptive trait that, for the most part, fails to cull us before reproductive age and so is invisible to natural selection. Bet you wish that one had drifted in you, huh?

The idea that dogs organize themselves into hierarchies is arguably the most pervasive in dog behavior. However, there is stunning discrepancy between the evidence to support this idea and its degree of popularity, and this to me is a fascinating question and one to which I'll return later.

Social Organization Models: A Mind Virus?

I recently read a dog training article in which the author asserts that dogs care about the order of exit through doorways. The indisputably popular notion that the dog charges through the doorway ahead of the owner to establish dominance is implausible to me. If it were true, though, this notion is certainly symptomatic of an

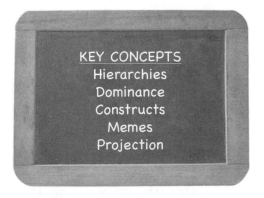

KEY CONCEPTS
Hierarchies
Dominance
Constructs
Memes
Projection

undesirable state of affairs (dog thinks he can dominate owner). Yet people choose to believe it. It seems that the more unbearable thought to some people is that they might be completely irrelevant, i.e., the dog is not considering the owner at all in the presence of an open door to the outdoors. To dominance fans, in other words, even when things are not as they should be (dog is dominating owner), the dog's behavior is at least in relation to them.

In her outstanding paper "A Struggle for Dominance—Fact or Fiction," Susan Friedman, professor of applied behavior analysis and parrot aficionado, addresses the use of dominance as explanation for (from our perspective) misbehavior of parrots. For example, are parrots that don't step up to be returned to their cages exerting dominance over their owners or do they just prefer to not go back into their cages and so engage in behaviors—notably aggression—that work to that end? Sound familiar, dog people?

Friedman points out that dominance is a construct, an inference about how or why an animal behaves as it does. And while constructs can be efficient chunking devices for constellations of behavior, they can also retard true understanding. They are "tightly bound by our own genetic, cultural and personal perspective. For most of us, thinking outside the proverbial 'box' to truly understand a child, spouse or friend is tough enough. Thinking outside one's own taxonomic [order] is an extraordinary challenge." Constructed explanations are also not falsifiable. This is especially true of dominance where any observation that contradicts a particular model can be explained away with a new, just-so addendum. For example, if in a supposed linear hierarchy a lower ranked dog is observed to get priority access to an important resource, dominance proponents will invoke a "temporary rank reversal," "order is in flux lately," or even "well, he's not feeling well today" clause to protect the system. And this pre-supposes that all observations that contradict the system are not filtered out in the first place!

In the absence of any research on social dominance in dogs, advocates borrow and expand from the captive wolf world. Expand is perhaps an understatement given the various discrepant spins on dog social systems, some of which I now list. Depending on which dog guru's book you read or which popular seminar you attend, you will be told that dogs form:

1. linear dominance hierarchies wherein order is maintained by superiors actively exerting rank (e.g. pinning, bullying, standing over) over subordinates

2. linear subordinance hierarchies wherein order is maintained by displays of appeasement by subordinates toward their superiors

3. non-transitive hierarchies where relationships within any dyad (pair) is fixed but out of which no overall hierarchy can be built

4. contextual dominance arrangements in which the nature of a disputed resource determines who wins

5. amorphous tiers of animals, where some are content with lowly status and others have dominant character traits (and

so fight a lot); from the ranks of the latter group a clear alpha emerges

6. across sex or separate sex variations on any of the above
7. hierarchies that include humans (or not)

Bear in mind, there is no evidence for any of these (with one exception, Ian Dunbar's unpublished bone dyad tests in the 1970's). A lazily-executed, informal search on Google will yield scores of research papers on cheetah reproductive physiology, hundreds on woodpecker foraging strategies, and thousands on ant social behavior, so you'd think there'd be roomfuls on dog hierarchies given the abandon with which we employ dominance to explain behavior and develop modification strategies. But I suspect the ground for Build Your Own Catchy Social Hierarchy System is rendered more fertile by the impressive evidence void.

Ah, but what about wolves?! Everybody knows that wolves form linear hierarchies (except when they don't!). In wolves, as in any non-domesticated species, social dominance is useless unless it confers reproductive advantage. A spectacular example with actual support is elephant seals, wherein male size results in victory over other males, which in turn pays off with near monopoly of a harem of females in a given season. The size of male elephant seals has been ratcheted up by this high stakes arms race. Among dog people then, not surprisingly, it is a well-worn dictum that the alpha pair are the exclusive breeders in a wolf pack (except when they're not), get first crack at carcasses (except when they don't), and lead the pack in its various activities.

Here's the rub. In a wild wolf pack, the "alpha" pair are parents in a nuclear family. They breed because they are socially mature adults. They are dominant over their offspring because parents can be said to be "dominant" over their children. Professor L. David Mech has researched wild wolves across the globe for nearly forty years and I had the pleasure of chatting with him in Minnesota last year. He is perplexed by the love affair with dominance among wolf people given that offspring in a wolf pack, if they live, inevitably reach reproductive age, disperse in order to find mates, reproduce and start their own packs. In all his years of research, he never saw an animal fail to reproduce if it lived long enough, making all wolves "alphas" once they mate.

Mech fears that some of his own early writings on wolves have fanned the dominance flames and many of these writings are no longer under his control and so continue to be published unrevised even though they do not reflect his thinking after a lifetime of research. He has published papers debunking dominance-as-trait, but this has yet to slow down dog people.

So why is dominance so hot? The answer might lie in human brains. In a 2002 paper published in *Nature Neuroscience*, Duke University researchers Scott Huettel, Beau Mack, and Gregory McCarthy found evidence of a brain module that compulsively seeks patterns whether there are actually any or not, and even when we have been made consciously aware that there are no patterns. In one experiment, subjects knew they were seeing random sequences of shapes, but their brains couldn't help but find "patterns." It could be that any perceived asymmetry in our dogs' win-loss records or dealings with other dogs will cause us to see a pattern such as, say, a hierarchy. And, any pattern that is (or is not) there usually prompts the search for explanations. Social dominance is one candidate and it has clearly hooked us, possibly for two reasons:

1. it is, I submit, a good model for explaining human social order and we project this readily to dogs (see Friedman, above)
2. it is a super-catchy idea, or "successful meme"

Memes are the cultural analogs of genes. They are ideas or pieces of information that are transmitted via imitation rather than via heredity. The single greatest criterion for meme success is the tendency to be repeated. Here is the interesting bit: notably absent from meme criteria is "that it is true." Urban legend transmission is among the most glaring examples and has been successfully modeled epidemiologically!

An idea can be so catchy that even when it is demonstrated to be false, it lives on. In other words, we protect catchy ideas, not true ideas. In one famous case, warnings about tattoos laced with LSD being given to children were admitted to be a hoax. The hook was too great, apparently, as one parent came back with a sarcastic "... thank you for pointing out that it is an urban legend. I'm sure all the drug dealers out there will be happy to hear that." Other parents acknowledged the hoax but, amazingly, carried on spreading it. A parents' newsgroup member wrote: "Parents aren't necessarily concerned with truth. We are concerned with our children's safety."

It is incredibly fascinating to me that were it ever convincingly proven that dogs are, well, just not as into dominance as we thought, the mind virus just might live on and on and on.

Neonate Puppies—What's Going On In There?

Dear Jean,

I've been in dogs for many years and have noticed a trend toward earlier and earlier socialization and training of puppies. The best time to start training used to be age six months. Then it went down to three months. Now I'm hearing that "it's over" by the time the puppy is three months old.

KEY CONCEPTS
Developmental periods
Neonatal
Transitional
Socialization
Plasticity

Most people do not even acquire their puppy before two months, which leaves precious little time. How can it "be over" by three months? Is this a myth? What are puppies capable of and at what age?

Early dog development has been divided into various periods. These discrete envelopes were proposed for our convenient identification and classification; the actual developmental process is, of course, continuous. The periods are: neonatal, transitional, and socialization.

The neonatal period begins at birth and extends until approximately fourteen days. The abilities and deficits of neonate puppies are well researched. Neonates, aside from having a well-developed sucking reflex, can do the following things on their own: crawl (not walk), distress vocalize, respond to tactile stimuli, and right themselves if they tumble onto their backs (my colleague Janis Bradley affectionately refers to them as being more like cockroaches than turtles in this regard). Conspicuously absent are the abilities to maintain a steady body temperature and to eliminate solo. Although destined to be thermoregulatory pros once adult, as are all mammals and birds, young puppies require careful attention to the temperature around them. They can do a little for themselves by spreading out when too warm and heaping together when cold, but that's it. And so exposure is too common a cause of neonate mortality.

Most neonates will urinate and defecate only in response to tactile stimulation. This is part of a system they co-evolved with their mothers. When the dam licks the puppies, they eliminate and the dam then eats the products. The result is the maintenance of a nest that is more hygienic and less conspicuous to predators. Interestingly, in spite of the relaxation of selection pressure for this system by domestication (i.e., most dogs without the trait still get hygiene support from human care-takers), it persists in most dogs. Compared to other can't-do-without-in-a-wild-context traits such as carcass dissection or food guarding, both of which have drifted significantly in domestic dogs and so are present in some individuals but not all, the nest-maintenance system is a curious hanger-on. It could be that litters are on their own enough of the time to render the system still valuable.

Following the neonatal period is the transitional period, which lasts until both the eyes and ears are open, usually by around age three weeks. Puppies in this fourteen to twenty-one day age range still have a relatively mask-like expression. They can stand and sometimes take a few faltering steps. Fascinatingly, it has been demonstrated that they can learn through reinforcement at this age. The mind runs amok with visions of itsy bitsy sits and downs in exchange for access to mom or a lap of liver infused milk. It could be, by the way, that neonates can also learn through reinforcement, however it has not yet been authoritatively proven.

The transitional period transitions to the much-talked-about socialization period. This is considered to be a sensitive period where experiences can have profound and lifetime effects on the puppy. Specifically, the puppy is forming a catalog of targets for social bonding. There is a convincing body of research that demonstrates that puppies that are not exposed to people during this period end up with severe and possibly refractory fearfulness of humans. It is therefore vital that puppies are socialized. There is not perfect agreement about what the cut-off age to achieve this is. Proposed ends to the socialization period range from eleven weeks to eighteen weeks. Some experts have suggested that there may be different envelopes for different breeds. However, as you point out, there is very good consensus that one gets better bang for their buck socialization-wise, the earlier one starts, regardless of the official end of the socialization period.

Exploiting Early Plasticity

Most puppies are not in the hands of owners until age seven weeks or more. Breeders, therefore, play an incredibly important role. Ian Dunbar has suggested that a primary criterion for breeder selection be the location where the litter is whelped. He would like to see all litters reared in a relatively high traffic area of the home, such as the kitchen or family room. No kennels, no garages, no back rooms. The reason for this is the benefit of constant passive exposure to household sights and sounds: kitchen appliance noises, conversation, TV, people walking around, vacuum cleaner, etc. from day one. Dunbar has also urged puppy buyers to be smart shoppers and request quantification of socialization efforts from breeders, i.e., how many new people per day the puppies have met and in what demographic categories. If the number is low (e.g. the family members and a few friends or neighbors), move on.

Another intriguing snippet of research that points to ultra-early intervention is the work of Carmen Battaglia on early puppy stimulation. He found that neonates that received mild, specific tactile stimuli on a daily basis grew up to be more stress resilient as adults. This finding begs for replication and an expanded research effort to determine exactly what breeders could be doing to further optimize early environment for the puppies they produce.

As far as training, there is a lack of research regarding optimal ages to start—or cut-off ages to complete—various tasks. In spite of this there is still a strong and fairly widely held feeling that earlier is better. It's been demonstrated that puppies aged two to three weeks can learn so the ideal starting age may creep downwards even more

from the current "begin the day you bring your puppy home."
Once again, this points to the vital role of breeders in the education
of puppies.

Puppy classes for puppies aged seven to eleven weeks are gaining
momentum. I think two factors are driving this. One is the increasing sense of urgency to exploit the earlier-is-better dictum. And, if
those authorities that postulate an end to the socialization period
at twelve or fourteen weeks are correct, the urgency is even greater.
The other factor is the increasing evidence that the disease risk to
puppies attending classes is not as great as once feared. Epidemiolo-
gist and veterinary behaviorist R.K. Anderson and veterinarians
at Purdue University, among others, have gone on record that not
only do the behavioral benefits outweigh the risk of exposure to
pathogens in a puppy class, but that the disease risk of a properly
run puppy class has been overblown. A properly run class means:

1. All puppies are healthy and have had an initial vaccine
   against parvo, distemper and bordatella.

2. Puppies are not walked to class on the ground outside, where
   they may encounter feces of unknown quantity dogs.

3. The puppy class premises are kept clean.

The Owner Signature: How We Build Our Dogs

Dear Jean,

I have owned seven dogs from four different groups and every one of them has loved to swim. I didn't think anything of this until I got to talking about swimming with some other dog people. All of them had some dogs that loved swimming, but others that didn't. At first I figured my seven in a row was

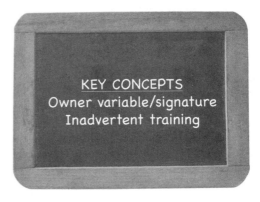

KEY CONCEPTS
Owner variable/signature
Inadvertent training

a fluke and then I got to thinking that every one of my seven dogs also loved the grooming table, jumped onto it when it was out, barked on command, and six out of seven put a paw on my foot to ask for a piece of scone when lying down next to me at Starbucks. I didn't deliberately try to train any of my dogs to do any of these things! A friend of mine has had five dogs (four different breeds from three groups) and all of them have had some sort of anxiety disorder. Although all these dogs I'm talking about are different from each other in so many ways, these uncanny similarities are starting to leap out at me. Is it my imagination or is the obvious common denominator—the owner—at the root here?

At a seminar over fifteen years ago Dr. Ian Dunbar said, "the owner variable is enormous." What he meant was that of all the factors that make up a dog's behavior—his genetics, puppy-hood, training, nutrition and health, and environment—the dog's daily interactions with the owner are extremely influential. I'd go one step further to include in the owner variable the owner's decisions about training, nutrition and health, and the dog's living situation. It's as though the owner puts a signature on the dog, and this is what I suspect you notice as that common denominator in the dogs you've owned.

Owner signatures can be overlooked because their features are easily ascribed to dog "personality," AKA genetics, or else watershed moments in early life such as traumas. While there is no question that both genetics and early trauma are big, never underestimate the small either, the day-to-day little things. Just as water can erode rock over time into canyons, micro-training day in and day out molds dog behavior.

For example, people vary in what they find amusing or endearing in dogs. Person one might laugh or clap when her puppy picks up a sock and runs around shaking his head. Person two might punish the dog and person three ignore him. Aside from any future likelihood of sock-directed behavior, there is also likely some mild effect on "picking things up" period or even "trying out a new behavior." There is no right or wrong answer here, just different ripples from different responses. Along with laughing or cheering, we smile at, attend to our dogs, and commence activities they like in a non-random way. Sometimes their behavior influences the timing of these events. When it does, expect there to be some gradual conditioning of behavior over time. You have apparently molded—inadvertently trained—all your dogs to put paws on your feet!

We humans also differ in the frequency with which we groom our dogs (and whether we make it fun for them as you have clearly done), walk our dogs, take them places that are fun for dogs, and take them to places that are usually less fun such as to veterinarians. This is partly dictated by necessity but also partly a function of someone's built-in tendency. For instance, compare any two dog owners and they will have different symptom thresholds that prompt them to bring their dog to the veterinarian. If a certain dog finds this a very stressful event and happens to belong to an owner who makes frequent trips, there will be an impact. Once again, this is not a value judgment—clearly people's decisions regarding veterinary care must be respected and clearly there are huge advantages to the better-safe-than-sorry philosophy. The point is that every single choice we make has ripples. All the ripples together are the owner signature. The fact that all your dogs were swimmers might be coincidence or it might be a reflection of where you often take your dogs and/or a testament to your skill or perseverance at teaching or encouraging swimming.

It can be interesting to watch owners with their dogs—at dog shows, dog parks, or anywhere dog owners congregate. Some tend to hustle their dogs along at the owner's choice pace, some patiently let their dogs sniff, and some vary depending on circumstances. A lifetime of any of these regimes will impact the dog's style of walking on leash. Some owners talk to their dogs a lot, some very little. Dogs whose owners talk to them all the time will have habituated much more to the sound of their owner's voice. They may also have doped out the nuances of certain words and intonation and how these are predictive of key dog-relevant events, both good and bad.

Some people get physically pushy, even violent with their dogs and others are much gentler. More ripples. Some people praise and baby-talk when their dogs are obedient and some when their dogs are cute (with the definition of "cute" in the eye of the beholder of course). If you poll a roomful of dog people and ask who has the cutest dog, most people will put up their hands. This is partly due to the fact that most people chose their dog and this choice is usually at least partly based on "chemistry," the technical term for "s/he's cute" or "this breed is cute." But the other part is the months and years of daily (inadvertent mostly) reinforcement for behaviors that are, from the owner's perspective, cute.

It's difficult to say whether your friend's dogs with the anxiety problems are partly the way they are because of your friend's signature on them. Such trends are a good springboard for introspection, however. We can all observe our dogs for evidence of our unique owner signatures.

What Is Play?

Dear Jean,

We added a beautiful Golden Retriever, Danny, to our family in the summer and we quite adore him. The only thing that concerns us is the manner in which Danny "plays" with other dogs—both at the dog park and with my sister's dog, Phoebe. He shows his teeth sometimes, growls a great deal, and bites the necks of the other dogs. We had him neutered, as per our contract with his breeder, and it made no difference. Then, at a litter reunion on his first birthday, he played with his littermates the same way! Our breeder said it was perfectly normal, but this is our first dog and I can tell you, it doesn't look the slightest bit normal to me. He has always played this way. At puppy class, when we were alarmed that he might be bullying other puppies, the instructor would have us hold him briefly and, inevitably, the other pup would, given the opportunity to escape, come back to him for more! Clearly we're not reading his play very well. Are you sure this is normal?

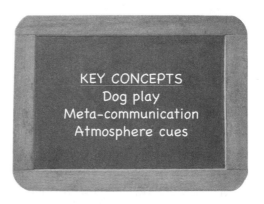

KEY CONCEPTS
Dog play
Meta-communication
Atmosphere cues

Play is one of the most interesting behaviors, yet is a poor cousin in the animal behavior world, viewed as more frivolous and less worthy of serious research grant money than, say, reproduction and eating. Luckily, what is understood about play addresses your concerns about Danny.

When dogs play, they borrow behaviors from other more goal-oriented activities—fighting, fleeing, hunting, and courtship—and jumble them all together, sometimes with key modifications. What's even more fascinating than the question of how you or I can tell it's play, is how the dogs can tell it's play, given that play consists of things like biting, body-slamming, jaw-wrestling with flashing toothy displays, chasing, pinning, and mounting! The answer lies in those key modifications and in what's called meta-communication. The two critical modifications to the "four F's" (fighting, fleeing, feeding and courtship) are:

1. Punches are pulled—behaviors such as slamming, pinning and, most notably, biting, are delivered with attenuated force.

2. Roles are frequently reversed—dogs take turns being biter and bitee, chaser and chasee, and being on the top and bottom in wrestling bouts. Note that role reversals can diminish if dogs that play together extremely frequently get into a "play rut," which is not worrisome if both parties are consenting.

The result of this self-handicapping is that during play you will regularly see a larger, stronger dog spending time "pinned" on the bottom, allowing himself to be bitten, and fighting and biting back with reduced intensity.

Meta-communication, or meta-signaling, is the other feature of play that distinguishes it from its goal-directed counterparts. A meta-communication is a message that qualifies other behaviors that come before and after it. It's the dog's way of saying "I'm about to bite, chase, snarl, and body-slam you, but it's just play." Ian Dunbar calls them "atmosphere cues" because of the tone, or atmosphere, that they set. Meta-signals are necessary because of the ambiguity of play behaviors. The meta-signals dogs use include play-bows—front quarters down, rear up, play face—an unmistakable open, wild-eyed, grinning expression; and exaggerated movements like inefficient, bouncy, rocking horse gaits, and unnecessary dekes to the side. Contrast this with a dog chasing a squirrel—efficient, flat-out running, not gamboling.

When meta-signaling, self-handicapping, and role-reversals slip too low or are not present at all, play doesn't look right, seeming to heat up and becomes overly intense. The dog whose play lacks these features may look like a broken record, repeating the same thing over and over, seemingly oblivious to the unwelcome effect it's having. The dog on the receiving end might at first continue to try to play normally but soon becomes distressed and signals "please stop" or "back off." If the dog with the play skill deficit does not read or respect this signal, fisticuffs may ensue, or bullying if the receiver opts not to defend. Such dogs may have adequate play histories, so it seems to not be an experiential deficit. Pit Bulls are over-represented among dogs with this play style, so I surmise a genetic component. These players can be reformed by teaching them to break off before they heat up and, once they are able to do so, abruptly terminating their opportunity to play when they fail to heed warnings to break off.

Danny does not sound like he is in this category. The acid test, if you're unsure, is the one your puppy class instructor did: restrain the presumed bully and see what the presumed victim does once free to escape. I would also suggest that while you're watching Danny play, count the number of times you observe full or partial play-bows, play face, and bouncy movements. It's clear from the history that he is doing an exemplary job inhibiting the force of his bites.

This pulling of punches is one of the conundrums of understanding the function of play. Why do animals play? Most mammals and many birds are believed to play and the behavior is not cheap—it takes time and energy, risks injury and, in the case of prey species, reduces vigilance as well as making them more conspicuous to predators. Considering these costs, there must be off-setting benefits. The leading contender among theories of the function of play is that it is some sort of rehearsal of the behaviors it borrows from.

Animals play most as juveniles and the type of play uncannily resembles key adult behaviors. For instance, predatory species like dogs, bite and chase a lot during play, and prey species like deer play escaping games. Male deer also play head-butting. Male sea lion pups bite five times more often than females. All this points to the rehearsal theory, but there are a couple of snags. One is that the pulling of punches, role-reversal, and inefficiency that make play play, also make it a poor means of combat rehearsal or prey killing. And, according to research to date, depriving juvenile animals of play does not seem to compromise their ability to function as adults, notably to perform the behaviors play is alleged to be rehearsing. We are talking about a paltry amount of research, however, and it is possible that tiny amounts of play are enough to confer benefit. But then, if tiny amounts are enough, why do so many species pay the higher cost of heftier amounts of play? The mystery of the function of play is yet to be unraveled but, in the meantime, we can enjoy watching dogs who are so masterful at it!

Dog Cognition Research

Dear Jean,

How smart are dogs, really?

If you ask most owners, they'll assure you their dogs are very smart indeed. And they would not be far off. But dogs, like most animals, are specialists. Dogs are in fact terrific examples of how it is more useful to think of

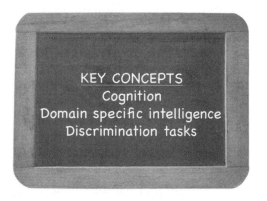

KEY CONCEPTS
Cognition
Domain specific intelligence
Discrimination tasks

intelligence in terms of specific brainpower domains rather than as a notion of "general intelligence," the stuff that IQ tests purport to measure in you and me. In their strong domains, dogs are up there. Stellar. In others, not so much.

First the talents. Dogs can estimate the passage of time with astounding accuracy. Not only do they know what time dinners and walkies are, they know whether it's Agility class night or not. Dogs are also masterful at noticing small cues in their environments to tip them off about what's going on. Ever noticed that your dog has learned that you turning the TV off at night means the next thing is bed time, and so trundles off unbidden? Whereas TV turn-off on Saturday afternoon is more ambiguous. Could be walkies. Could be car-rides. Could be nothing. Has your dog doped out that keys plus briefcase equal the abyss of solitude for a few hours whereas the same keys plus a "Chuckit™" mean nirvana at the dog park? Does your dog know the road's turn-off to the dog park? The one to the groomer? There's a Border Collie in Germany that can discriminate 200 different words (all, amazingly, variations on the theme of "tennis ball").

People underestimate dogs' ability to do fine discriminations all the time. It's a well-worn myth that one shouldn't give a dog an old shoe to chew lest he learn to chew all shoes. It might actually be tricky to teach a dog a category like "shoe," given that shoes might be leather, fabric, rubber, have laces or not, be light, strappy and open, or weigh several pounds. Humans are very good at this kind of classification by function or other high concept. Dogs are less about headings and more about specific case. It's a no-brainer for a dog to learn that this shoe here is his to dissect at will, but those leather goods on the racks in the closet and the ones on the entryway mat? Strictly verboten. I know dog trainers that, for kicks, teach their dogs to discriminate US currency by scent. I have difficulty discriminating US currency at all.

Recent research has demonstrated that dogs read human gestures more readily than both chimpanzees and wolves. Even kennel-reared dogs outperformed hand-reared wolves, suggesting that the capacity is not a product of lots of experience around people. Part of dogs' specialization is clearly making the most of their human-rich environment. It's also been suggested by a study that dogs gauge their play solicitations to other dogs based on whether the potential playmate is attending or not. Dog behavior researcher Marc Bekoff points out that dogs are clearly by no means "dumbed down wolves."

There's no way to—pardon the pun—intelligently discuss cognition without drawing the distinction between what has been scientifically proven and what most people believe based on interpretations of their own day to day experience with dogs. This topic tends to leave people cold, as though science rains on some sort of confabulation parade. But the (very interesting) fact of the matter is, there is enormous discrepancy in key areas between what people think dogs are good at and what dogs are actually good at as soon as other explanations are ruled out. It's why we love science so. Let me give you an example.

I doubt there's a day that goes by wherein a dog trainer somewhere is not regaled by an owner about how his dog imitates. This dog imitates that dog. The puppy imitated the resident adult. The dog imitated the owner, the cat, or the budgie. Poll dog owners, even dog fanciers, and they will tell you, yes, dogs can imitate. One dog peed. Then the other one did. See? Or the more sophisticated version: one dog opened the latch, broke into the yard, and terrorized the ducks. Then the other dog did it. First time ever. See?

The sticky thing is that many processes can account for an animal seeming to do something after witnessing a model, not just imitation. And, as soon as conditions are controlled so that those other means are not available, dogs suddenly can't "imitate." Imitation is defined as an animal replicating the behavior of another animal after one viewing. The behavior can't be a fixed action pattern such as barking, urinating, chasing something, etc. Many such behaviors are readily socially facilitated—triggered in a non-imitative way, or ratcheted up in intensity—in dogs. Right off the bat many imitation anecdotes are out of the running. There can't be enhancement of a key spot or thing via intense activity: does witnessing random but intense and apparently successful activity of a model dog at the latch help as much as witnessing a skillful latch manipulator dog? If it does, it's not imitation. Such "two-action tests" are the current gold standard for inferring imitation and dogs are so far unimpressive at them. The behavior must be novel to make the criteria for imitation. And learning processes such as operant conditioning must be ruled out. Bottom line: in spite of some effort to find evidence of imitation in dogs, researchers so far have come up empty-handed. So, if dogs can imitate, there is a global canine conspiracy to keep science in the dark about it.

Now, that said, there are some intriguing whiffs of proto-imitation in the dog cognition research. For example, if you put a dog behind a fence, put a toy on the other side and demonstrate one of two possible detours around the fence, the dog is more likely than chance to take the detour you showed him. Which brings us back to domain-specific talents. This detour copying is imitative, no doubt about it. But it's limited to this domain: route-taking. Dogs don't have the all-purpose imitate-anyone-doing-anything module we humans take for granted. To me, this is the heart of the divide between what science tells us dogs can (and can't) do and what people continue to insist they can. Imitation comes so incredibly readily to us that we can't imagine a mind that can't do it. We especially can't imagine a familiar mind that can't do it. And, given that humans are capable of ascribing agency to cartoon sponges, it's not surprising that our theory of mind module runs amok when it comes to those most splendid of surrogate children, our dogs. They are very, very like us. They bond readily and strongly. They feel palpably similar emotions. They are fabulous consequence learners. Their proto-theory-of-mind module seems able to dope out whether another dog is attending or not. So when they appear to do something that we would have done via imitation, we project imitative ability.

Ambivalence and Conflicting Motivation

Dear Jean,

My Afghans know when it's bath day—as soon as I start assembling the towels and prepping the tub, they go into a funk. If I'm not mistaken, this is due to classical conditioning. Anyway, as my husband strolled by before bath time this afternoon, he remarked that I was "boring Arnold to death" because he saw him yawn. There is no way this dog was bored. Was this a calming signal, redirected behavior, or just pure stress?

KEY CONCEPTS
Classical conditioning
Displacement behaviors
Conditioned reinforcers
Calming signals
Redirected behavior
Conflict

Yes, good call about the classical conditioning—the anticipation of baths based on the pre-bath stimuli is absolutely textbook. The interpretation of yawning opens up a most interesting kettle of fish. And you're also right here—it's not boredom.

The leading explanation for Arnold's yawning is that it was a displacement behavior. This is an action that pops out when an animal is in conflict about how to respond to something. In this case, he might have been in conflict about whether to flee, fight the bath, or simply give up and allow it. The conflict produces low-grade stress and this can manifest as a behavior with no relevance or relation to the context.

Have you ever noticed dogs yawning during sit-stays, in vet waiting rooms, or when they're slightly worried about something? Displacement. You may also have seen a cat stalking a bird, rush and narrowly miss catching it, and then suddenly groom himself. This would also likely be classified as a displacement behavior. The minor stress secondary to the thwarted hunting attempt fuels displacement grooming. (Many people, naturally, think the cat is embarrassed and trying to act "casual.")

Displacement behaviors are often self-directed: animals might groom or rub themselves, and humans scratch their heads when confused or solving a problem. An interesting study on chimpanzees a few years ago demonstrated that as they were given progressively more difficult problems to solve, the chimpanzees engaged in more and more self-directed behaviors. But, if they were given auditory cues to let them know they were on the right track (conditioned reinforcers, in effect!), the self-directed behaviors were reduced. This suggests that positive feedback reduces the stress of solving a problem.

You asked whether Arnold's yawn might have been a calming signal. If I understand calming signals correctly, they are communications to other animals. Like appeasement gestures, they have as their objective to inhibit aggression in the other animal. A case could possibly be made that what would normally be classified as a simple displacement behavior may have signaling value or intention in some instances. But in other cases, the case is too weak as there is nobody around to signal to. The behavior quite predictably pops out when the animal is stressed or worried, period. So, I'd say beware of over-interpretation here.

Displacement behavior is not quite the same as redirected behavior. Redirected behavior is an action that fits the context well but is performed toward an alternative target. If a dog is highly motivated to attack another dog, but is prevented by his leash from doing so, he may bite the leash or even his handler. Two dogs agitating behind a fence at a passer-by might unload their frustration on each other. Contrast this with displacement activities, which are performed at the right target (i.e., grooming oneself) but at the "wrong" time (when in conflict). So, to summarize:

> Displaced behavior = right target, wrong time
> Redirected behavior = right time, wrong target

The types of conflict that generate both these types of behavior also vary. Conflicts can be internal—within the animal—or between the animal and its environment. Let's look at internal conflicts first. A psychologist by the name of Kurt Lewin was the first to examine internal conflicts experimentally. He divided these into three main types:

1. Approach-approach conflicts, where two equally or nearly equally attractive goals beckon the animal at the same time. For example, in a Premack recall exercise, where a distracter holds tasty food in an enclosed hand while the empty-handed owner calls the dog from a few feet away—the dog must move away from the food "magnet" in order to collect it— dogs frequently bark. This could be an approach-approach conflict between going to the owner (which presumably has been reinforcing in the past) and leaving an apparent "bird in the hand." It could also be pure thwarting (see below).

2. Avoidance-avoidance conflicts (or dilemmas), where one must choose between two rotten options. A good dog example is coercing a fearful dog to hold a stay in order to be patted. If the dog breaks, he is corrected. If he stays, he is patted by someone he's afraid of. This kind of conflict can wreak havoc with an animal's body.

3. Approach-avoidance conflicts, where the same stimulus or goal attracts and repels at the same time. This third type is also familiar to dog people. Dogs that are simultaneously curious and afraid of something will do stretch-investigations or oscillate between approach and withdrawal. Barking and whining—displacement behaviors—are also commonly seen in these conflicting motivation situations.

External conflicts are between constraints imposed by the external environment and the animal's motivation. This is known as thwarting. Unlike internal conflicts, in thwarting scenarios the animal's motivational ducks are in a row, but the behavior the animal has "decided" upon is physically impossible. Imagine, for instance, making an authoritative decision to flee a predator but having your leg caught under a rock. Very stressful, but in a different way from having a hard time making a decision. Barrier frustration is the most common dog example.

Konrad Lorenz also had a well known take on displacement activities. They fit well into his hydraulic model of behavior. He submitted that "action-specific energy" was a force inside the animal and that it accumulated over time. Dogs might, for example, build up "play energy," "chasing energy," or "barking energy." When enough specific energy had built up, an animal would feel generally more energized. If it encountered an environmental trigger that corresponded to a particular filled-up reservoir, a fixed action pattern would be released.

If, according to Lorenz, energy had built up in the reservoirs for more than one action and the animal encountered triggers for two opposing behaviors, energy would overflow and a displacement behavior could be released. You can see how this mirrors the approach-avoidance conflict model. Two "drives" kick in simultaneously. Lorenz also postulated that "vacuum behaviors"—the appearance of a fixed action pattern without its characteristic trigger—are the result of overflowing specific reservoirs.

Nutrition and Behavior

Dear Jean,

Nutrition is a hot but complicated topic. It's touted as having a role in everything from resolving or managing health issues to optimal condition. But aside from performance diets for working dogs, interest seems confined to the effects of food on the body, rather than on behavior. Is anything

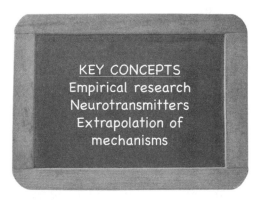

KEY CONCEPTS
Empirical research
Neurotransmitters
Extrapolation of
mechanisms

known about how the diet of dogs affects, or might affect, their behavior?

The "affects or might affect" wording in your question is very important. It points to the two different bases for fiddling with nutrition in dogs with a view to improving behavior. One is empirical research: well-controlled studies on the effects on behavior of manipulating diet components or supplementation in dogs. When dogs—or a subgroup of dogs, such as those with a certain behavior problem—consume X amount of substance Y, Z change in behavior is measurable. Then, when a reliable, replicable effect is found, mechanisms will be proposed: how and why does this manipulation exert an effect? Because there is a lot known about biochemical mechanisms, this can direct further research efforts to increase and refine knowledge of empirical effects.

Which brings us to the second source for gleaning insights about nutrition and behavior: known mechanisms. Because the empirical research on nutrition and behavior in dogs is so incredibly scarce, we're left speculating about interventions that might plausibly exert an effect based on what's known about food, supplements, and the brain. This is much, much weaker, in my opinion, than a bona fide empirical result, but at the very least this approach can suggest where research efforts could be directed. Also, in the absence of empirical knowledge, it could be argued that it's better than nothing in an individual case to play around with nutrition and supplements that are in the can't-hurt-might-help category.

Let's look at the empirical research first. Two studies, one in 1996 and one in 2000, tentatively concluded that low protein diets can reduce aggression. Both compared diets in the 17-18% protein range with diets in the 30-32% protein range. One study also looked at supplementing the amino acid tryptophan to the two diets and found that for aggression directed at the family, either the tryptophan addition or reduced protein, had a favorable impact, while both interventions were necessary to reduce aggression directed at strangers.

This is far from a slam dunk for the low protein connection. It raised consternation in the natural/raw food diet crowd, whose dogs routinely consume relatively high protein diets and who claim favorable effects on behavior from such a diet. As for empirical research, one study in 2002 found that a diet higher in digestible protein and fat reduced reactivity in shelter dogs. So much, much more needs to be done to clarify what's going on vis-a-vis dietary protein and aggression.

This is pretty much it as far as direct research on dog behavior and nutrition. There is, however, all kinds of interesting research on dietary components and the brain in a wide variety of species, including humans, performed in an attempt to increase understanding of human behavior and mental disorders. Are there grounds for inference from these studies for those of us in dog behavior? There might be. Dogs have been relatively popular animal models in human nutrition research over the years (unfortunately on other topics in nutrition than behavior) and so much is known about the validity of extrapolating results from dog to human subjects. It therefore holds water that we might be able to go the other way—from humans to dogs—in extrapolating results from research on diet, supplementation and human neurochemistry.

The Monoamine Connection

There are three types of neurotransmitters—chemical messengers—in the brain: large neuropeptides, such as beta-endorphins; and two kinds of smaller molecules, amino acids, such as GABA, the inhibitor molecule, and glutamate, the excitatory molecule, and, finally, monoamines. The monoamines, though small in percentage, are huge in influence. They have been strongly implicated again and again in affecting everything from violent behavior and impulsivity to compulsive behavior, anxiety, and depression. They may even be the master regulators of the amino acid neurotransmitters.

Monoamines come in four varieties: the catecholamines (notably dopamine and norepinephrine), acetylcholine, histamine (which promotes wakefulness—this is why anti-histamines can make you drowsy), and serotonin. They are synthesized from precursor molecules and then stored in vessicles in pre-synaptic neurons, the cells on the sending side of the gap between brain cells. Once released, they park in receptor sites on post-synaptic neurons, thus allowing communication between cells. Monoamines are then inactivated in two ways, either by being captured by re-uptake transporters to be stored in the pre-synaptic vessicles for next time, or else degraded into their constituents by monoamine oxidase enzymes.

A veritable cornucopia of medications has been developed to manipulate this system (see Understanding Psychotropic Medications in Section 4). It has also proven responsive to diet. For instance, the essential amino acid tryptophan is a precursor (building block) of serotonin, the monoamine most implicated in aggression, anxiety, and low impulse control. Research has shown that in rats and humans, a tryptophan deficient diet increases aggressiveness. Evidence like this along with the tryptophan supplementation and aggression study mentioned earlier suggests that precursor loading—the provision of extra building blocks of key neurotransmitters in the diet—could be an avenue worth exploring more in dogs. Tryptophan rich foods include turkey, grapefruit, bananas, and milk.

Measurable increases in serotonin can also be achieved by supplementing with 5-hydroxytryptophan (5-HTP), the intermediate molecule in the conversion of tryptophan to serotonin. There is division of opinion regarding whether it is advisable to also supplement vitamin B6 when taking 5-HTP, and whether an enzyme (decarboxylase) inhibitor should be taken to delay the conversion of 5-HTP to serotonin to the brain rather than it taking place predominantly in the bloodstream.

What about other neurotransmitters?

Precursor loading can also work to increase levels of our other favorite monoamines, acetylcholine and the catecholamines norepinephrine and dopamine. For instance, L-theanine, found in green tea, can produce a calming effect by increasing GABA and dopamine in the brain. Then there's phenylalanine, an amino acid that is converted to tyrosine, another amino acid, which is in turn converted into the catecholamines norepinephrine, and dopamine. Low levels of phenylalanine, tyrosine, norepinephrine and dopamine have all been associated with depression in humans. Rich sources of phenylalanine include chicken, turkey, fish, soy products, avocados, dairy products, and lima beans.

Dopamine and serotonin production could be stepped up by supplementing S-adenosylmethionine (SAM-e), especially if taken in conjunction with folate and vitamin B12. Large scale clinical efficacy trials (on humans) are currently being conducted on SAM-e in the US. It has already been shown to accelerate the action of tri-cyclic anti-depressants (such as Clomicalm and Elavil), one of the difficulties with which has been the lag (often up to six weeks or more) between commencing therapy and visible results. Wouldn't it be fabulous to see double blind placebo controlled clinical trials of SAM-e used in conjunction with tri-cyclics (and even the SSRI Prozac) for anxiety disorders and aggression in dogs?

Acetylcholine is the most abundant neurotransmitter in the brain and known to be involved in learning and memory. An important precursor to it is choline, one of the substances that make up lecithin, a fatty substance produced by the liver. Manufacture of lecithin requires B vitamins, essential fatty acids and magnesium, so successful choline supplementation requires a diet that includes these other nutrients.

Dimethylaminoethanol (DMAE) has been increasingly implicated in maintaining the health of aging brains, learning, memory, and even mood. It can be found in deep ocean fish such as sardines or in supplement form. It's best taken with vitamin B5.

The essential fatty acids are another promising avenue with regard to both healthy brain aging and psychiatric disorders. An English study is in progress, which is examining whether hostility in children can be reduced by increasing essential fatty acids. Low omega-3 fatty acid levels, relative to omega-6 and saturated fats, have already been associated with depression in humans. EFAs control enzyme systems and certain aspects of neurotransmitter function, so it's not a stretch to propose mechanisms.

One last nugget worth mentioning is a study that found one third of depressed human subjects had a food allergy compared with only 2% of the controls. If low-grade food allergies can manifest as mental symptoms, it could open up a significant avenue for dietary intervention to aid behavior problems dogs.

Malingering: Do Dogs Ever Fake It?

Dear Jean,

Do dogs feign illness or lameness to get out of doing something they don't want to do (or to get sympathy or attention)? I swear my Golden Retriever, Hannah, does this. If she doesn't want to do an exercise in obedience, she lies down and then seems to have difficulty getting up, as though

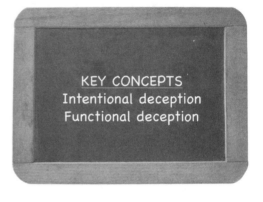

KEY CONCEPTS
Intentional deception
Functional deception

she were aching or tired. But if a squirrel were to run by, she suddenly is fine!

This is a fine and fascinating can of worms that you open. Let's discuss a little of what's known about deception in animals, including humans, and then circle back to Hannah's behavior. First, a human example. Linda's office is having a party and she would like her husband, Joey, to attend it with her. On the afternoon before the party, Joey complains of not feeling well. Linda ends up going to the party on her own. While she is gone, Joey watches a football game.

What are the possible explanations for Joey's behavior? One is that he is ill. Another is that he actually feels okay but would prefer to not attend the party and behaves in a way to achieve that end. But it's even more complicated than that as there are two different ways he can actually achieve this deceptive end. One is that he thinks it through, that is, he represents the events, including their likely outcomes, in his head. "Hmm. I don't want to go, but reneging has social consequences. However, illness is something beyond my control that Linda would understand. It is also something I could feign well enough to deceive her, and everybody would win: she gets to go the party, I get to stay home, and her feelings aren't hurt." After playing some version of this plan out in his head, he enacts it. This is intentional deception: the plan is mentally explored and a decision made before behavior—even novel behavior without any learning history (important)—occurs. Humans are very good at this. Dogs, not so much.

Now for deception option two. Joey may have a successful history of getting off such hooks via illness or appearing ill to others—no premeditation or intentionality, but a reinforcement history for certain behaviors in certain contexts. For instance, lying down, looking reluctant, talking about not feeling 100%, and other related behaviors may have delayed or prevented unpleasant consequences. Such behavior is infinitely trainable, in humans, dogs and oodles of other animals. Same outcome, different mechanism.

From an outsider's standpoint, it is not possible to tell what is going on from eyeballing Joey on the day of Linda's party. These mechanisms function to achieve the same end: Joey looks ill and doesn't attend the party. Only in intentional deception are there theoretical machinations in Joey's head, the mental playing out of the scenario in advance, the one which requires Joey to mentally represent events ahead of time. This is the one people usually find morally inferior. "Free will" and all that.

There is a lot of the other kind—functional deception—in the animal world. Birds do broken wing displays to lure predators from nests, possums play possum, cats get down low and stalk. Natural selection has shaped animals to do these things the same way a trainer and a clicker can shape a dog to crawl along like a commando, or reinforcement history shapes helpless or ill-seeming behaviors in people without their conscious awareness. The behavior works and so is selected for, in one case, by selecting successively approximating genes over millennia, in the other by selecting successively approximating behaviors in "real time." Neither requires the mental gymnastics of intentional deception.

So, to summarize: humans are very, very fluent at both evolved in or conditioned in (functional) deception and intentional deception (which is also, incidentally, an "evolved in" ability—everything, and I mean everything, is "evolved in"). We can also do hybrids. A behavior may be kicked off by a deliberate, intentional deception and then be conditioned by favorable consequences and get stronger. Or deception may be initially conditioned and, at some point, reach conscious awareness and at that point get refined or even self-punished. Or, an intentional deception that is not successful or punished by an outside agent gets reduced or dropped from your repertoire. Deception, you see, drives the evolution of counter-measures in others, resulting in an arms race of sophistication, which is part of why people have "he's lying" radar as well as some fancy lying abilities (including, interestingly, the ability to self-deceive to camouflage lying flags!). Arms races are compelling selection pressures in nature. Leopard spots and the urge to station themselves downwind is driven by gazelle eyesight, scenting ability and vigilance, which drive better spots, and so on.

Dogs, on the other hand, while masterful at being conditioned to behave in ways that function to get them off hooks, cannot perform intentional deception the way you and I can. What this means is that Hannah has likely been successful in the past at ending obedience training or certain exercises with certain behaviors that you interpret as malingering. But just because you can do it with intentionality doesn't mean she can.

This raises some questions. The most interesting one to me is why people persist in believing dogs can intentionally deceive the way humans can in spite of substantial evidence to the contrary. That there are other ways to achieve the same goal seems to rub many people the wrong way.

I think this is because we have profound difficulty imagining different minds. And we furthermore value or rank animals according to how similarly their minds are to ours! It is the brain judging equivalent to evaluating your dog's conformation based on a breed standard consisting of human movie actors. We readily appreciate dog bodies relative to dog standards, but when it comes to cognition, the gold standard is inevitably human. Ironically, part of what makes it difficult for us to imagine minds that are not like ours is evolutionary pressure that drove our minds to be able to represent other minds like ours. A significant element in the early environment of humans was the minds of other humans, an arms race of Machiavellian navigation. Fast forward to today. Dogs are family members and so are subject to fast and loose anthropomorphism.

Another question this raises is why on earth Hannah doesn't want to do obedience? A careful re-examination of how you are motivating her may be in order. Finally, I would like to point out that it is entirely possible that Hannah does have a bona fide physical problem. Dogs with pain or infirmity routinely rise to hyper-motivating occasions such as squirrels, so her apparent ability to suddenly get up or appear athletic may simply mean she's toughing out a real problem when sufficiently motivated. Squirrels are up there. Part of your job may turn out to be getting obedience up there.

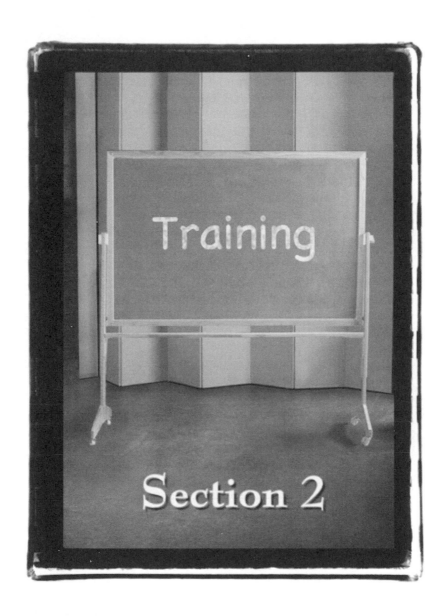

Training

Section 2

Dog Training Philosophies

Dear Jean,

I watched a program on "The Dog Whisperer." It sounded like the training was based on projecting the right "energy," but it looked like collar correction training. Which is it?

KEY CONCEPTS
Operant conditioning
Reinforcement
Punishment
Aversives
Obfuscation of motivators

There is perhaps no hotter topic in dog training than philosophy: how exactly does one get the job done. There are two ways to examine philosophy. One is to objectively observe what the trainer does, especially as far as the provision of consequences—events that occur after behavior —and then look at the result on the behavior's frequency. What is consequence X and does it make behavior Y increase or decrease in frequency? This is then classified into the quadrants of operant conditioning.

The other way to look at training philosophies is to record the rhetoric used by the trainer herself. What does the dog trainer say she is doing? The final and most interesting part is to then compare what the trainer says she is doing with what she is actually doing.

Let's look at objective classification first. Many dog trainers don't think they are employing some subset of the four types of operant conditioning. But, I contend that they inevitably are and that this is the most informative way to break down philosophy. The four quadrants in operant conditioning are:

1. Positive reinforcement: the initiation of something, which increases the frequency of the behavior it immediately follows.

2. Negative punishment: the terminating of the same stuff as in #1, i.e., the removal of something which decreases the frequency of the behavior it immediately follows.

3. Negative reinforcement: the terminating of something, which increases the frequency of the behavior that termination immediately follows.

4. Positive punishment: the initiation of the same stuff as in #3, i.e., the introduction of something which decreases the frequency of the behavior it immediately follows.

For all animals, food, water, and sex function as positive reinforcers. This is because if they don't find food and water reinforcing they die. You can also put your money on sex as a positive reinforcer because all organisms that we routinely train are descended from a nearly billion year unbroken line that had sex at least once. That's a pretty good genetic track record, so it's a reasonable inference that any given individual will have inherited the trait.

By extension, the termination of food, water, and sex, or the loss of opportunities to gain them, will all function as negative punishers. My favorite negative punishment example comes from chicken camp, where dog trainers go to sharpen up their skills by training chickens. One of the tasks is a visual discrimination. A cardboard triangle, square, and circle are put down and the chicken is reinforced for pecking the triangle. The chicken is highly motivated as it is on a closed economy (100% of the food ration is earned in training), so triangle pecking spikes dramatically in frequency. The training periods are usually two minutes long and there may be only half a dozen or so in one day. So each two minute opportunity to earn food is important to the chicken.

Here's the negative punishment part. If the chicken pecks the square or the circle, not only is it not reinforced with food, it's punished by removal of the triangle, let's say for thirty seconds. So for thirty seconds out of its two minute training period, the chicken can't peck the triangle, its only gateway to earning food reinforcement. What this results in is a chicken who is both hot to peck the triangle and extremely unlikely to touch the square or circle. Classic negative punishment.

Negative reinforcement is something many of us have experienced in the form of analgesia. Let's say you have a bad headache. You try painkiller brand number one to no avail. Then brand number two without luck. You then try brand number three and it relieves the headache. If the next time you have a headache you reach for brand three right away, you have experienced negative reinforcement: the termination of the pain and the increase in the behavior—brand three ingestion—that accomplished that.

If you were careless walking down your basement stairs, banged your head and that is what gave you the headache in the first place, you might avoid those stairs in the future or avoid walking down them carelessly. This would be positive punishment. Note that the same aversive stimulus—the headache—functions as positive punishment when it starts and as negative reinforcement when it ends, just as the chicken's food can function as both positive reinforcement when it starts and negative punishment when it is removed.

In dog training, food, toys (for some dogs), access to other dogs or the owner (especially after an absence), and patting and praise are all things that some trainers use as positive reinforcers by providing them to increase the frequency of behaviors like coming when called, sitting, walking nicely on leash, eliminating in the right place, and chewing the right stuff. Some dog trainers also employ these things in their role as negative punishers by terminating them to decrease behaviors like playing roughly, jumping up, and breaking stays. This represents one objective philosophical divide: the use of positive reinforcement and/or negative punishment. There are also mini divides with regard to reinforcer type: some trainers employ certain reinforcers, but object to the use of others. For instance, praise and patting are used, but not food. Other trainers use whatever works.

Aversives are things that signal to an animal imminent bodily injury or death—in other words, they're painful or scary. In dog training, the most common aversive stimuli are collar jerks, throwing items at the dog, shaking him, pinning him on his back, loud noises, hitting him, spraying him with water or with a chemical such as citronella, pinching his ear, and electric shock. Just as with the initiating and terminating of food, toys, play, etc., these aversives can be started and stopped. And, as with some positive reinforcers, there is a range of potency from dog to dog. Some dogs are sensitive, finding a wide variety and intensity of attempted aversives painful or scary, while other dogs are much tougher.

So another divide among dog trainers is whether they employ aversives and, to a lesser degree, whether they employ them as positive punishers to decrease unwanted behavior, as negative reinforcers to increase desired behaviors (such as an ear-pinch retrieve), or both.

If you videotape a trainer in action and count the (hopefully well-timed) consequences she supplies and then note the effect of these on the frequency of responses, you can calculate which operant quadrants she uses and how often. A trainer might be 72% positive reinforcement and 28% negative punishment. Another trainer may be 55% positive punishment, 40% positive reinforcement and 5% negative reinforcement. And so on. This ratio may fluctuate depending on which dog is being trained to do (or not do) which behavior.

Now the fun part. If you then interview the trainer or read descriptions by the trainer of her training, you are unlikely to get percentages of operant quadrants utilized broken down by dog and/or behavior. Some trainers will deny they are using operant conditioning at all! Instead, the trainer might do one of three things:

1. Refer to dog cognitions and the effect on these of various interventions, most commonly their effect on an imagined social structure, such as "If you let the dog go through doorways ahead of you he will think he is the leader. Ensure you always go through first so he will see you as the leader."

2. Refer to the need to communicate to the dog in "dog language," either about social structures (see #1) or to be understood at all, such as "The mother dog expresses her disapproval to puppies by shaking them and growling, so mimic this by shaking your puppy and using a low, growly voice."

3. Employ language from psychotherapy models or mysticism, such as "Believing each dog is perfect at being that particular dog means every dog is treated as an individual. It is recognized that each is only capable of responding according to his or her specific and individual merits and limitations."

Of course, as none of these are verifiable, they could very well be true. So it could be that the trainer you observed on television is projecting energy. If the collar corrections are decreasing behavior, however, there is no doubt that he is employing positive punishment, perhaps as the sole "real" intervention or perhaps in conjunction with the energy projection.

History of the Hierarchy

A linear hierarchy was first described in chickens, resulting in the term "pecking order." In the 1930's and 40's, short-term studies of wolf packs were performed and these introduced similar ideas about hierarchies to help explain competition among wolves over resources such as food, mates, and choice sleeping locations.

What was not known at that time is that appeasing behaviors, which help solve conflicts by lessening an opponent's aggression, are willingly offered by the more submissive animal, not forced by the top dog. Also, long-term studies on wild wolf populations suggest a minor, if any role, for hierarchies (in contrast to the near obsession of captive wolf research with the concept!). And, interestingly, there is not one documented case of a normal mother wolf or dog "scruff-shaking" puppies.

In spite of the flimsy evidence, the concept of dominance was very catchy and trickled down over the years into the dog training culture. Dozens of books and methods sprung up that admonished owners to be "leader of the pack" (even though all existing evidence indicates that dogs don't form packs) and warned of the misbehavior that would ensue if the dog was allowed to assume the "alpha" position.

But the dominance concept continued to spread. Training methods that relied heavily on aversives such as pain and startle, to motivate the dog used dominance ideas to justify the harsh techniques—one needed to put the dog "in his place."

Think Leverage, Not Dominance

A more useful way to think about modifying dog behavior is in terms of leverage, rather than dominance. Paying attention to and taking control of what the dog wants—attention, walks, food, access to the yard, access to other dogs and smells on the ground, door opening services, play, etc.—and providing them for desired rather than undesired behavior—will achieve a well-trained dog as well as positive associations with both the training process and trainer.

Puritanism and Reward Training

A friend of mine recently adopted a very shy dog. Being a dog trainer, when he first met the dog, he did all the right things: let her come to him at entirely her own pace; never reached for her; and tossed, then hand fed her very high value food treats over and over. It didn't take long for the dog to not only warm up to him, but to fall in love, and hard. The look on this dog's face when she hears his voice or sees him coming could sell dog food.

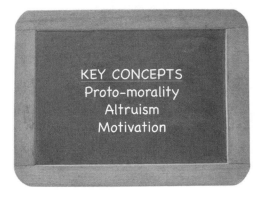

KEY CONCEPTS
Proto-morality
Altruism
Motivation

Conversely, the dog remained wary of, if not more fearful, of my friend's wife. My trainer friend laid out the desensitization and Pavlov style training that had so done the trick for him and his wife did a stellar job of not rushing things—but eschewed the baggie full of fabulous treats. When reminded to hand feed her at an opportune moment, she confessed, lamenting that, "I want her to love me for me, not because of the food."

For many, many people, it is not good enough (potentially corrupting in fact) for the dog to do what we'd like, to be obedient, polite, and friendly because of a well-executed reward history. He must do and feel what we'd like for the right reasons. Incisiveness regarding motive is such a pervasive feature of the human brand that we have a hard—no, wait, impossible—time imagining a mind without it.

We are nothing if not Machiavellian about the inner machinations of others. And it seems desperately important to many that the dog not only be well-behaved, but be well-behaved for no other reason than their (the owner's) wonderfulness or position at the apex of some imagined pecking order. Aside from the strong shades of narcissism, it's a training quagmire. Now proto-moral qualities, such as sense of fairness, have been demonstrated in chimpanzees, so we don't have a monopoly, but in dogs and their more closely related cousins have none, nothing, diddley-squat, zip. The complete absence in dogs of a complex morality wouldn't be a problem if our obsession with it didn't slow down the training cause.

In cases like my friend's wife, the holding out for grander motives will at best retard progress and at worst derail it altogether. Dogs are bonding animals and there is unquestionably a decent chance that the dog will, over time, both habituate to the woman and bond to her. Bonding is a trait at the intersection of the dog and human repertoires—we both do it in spades. But don't cue the music just yet. Fearful animals don't always go in this direction. Some spontaneously worsen with exposure. This is called sensitization. From a purely techie standpoint, it is a spin of the wheel in an area on which we best not gamble.

And before we get all biggety about bonding, recall that kidnap victims bond to their captors and people in abusive domestic situations remain bonded to their tormentors. Mistreated dogs are also unquestionably bonded to their ghastly owners, though their devotion is always tinged with fear and—to quote *Whole Dog Journal* editor Nancy Kearns—wary subservience. Less noble this part. So, based on the (if you think about it) slightly tortured logic of I-don't-want-to-give-rewards, an abuser must be some kind of paragon and the relationship he has with his victim the most august of all, as not only does it not get any turbo charging from rewards, but withstands rotten treatment. Hmm.

The other fallout of iron-fistedness about rewards is that it leaves one in a motivational void for anything other than cheap behaviors in non-distracting environments. Dogs, like all properly functioning living organisms, don't waste their behavioral dollar. There is no free lunch in animal training. In the words of applied behavior analyst Dr. Susan Friedman, "behavior doesn't flow like a fountain; behavior is a tool to produce consequences." This human craving for the appearance of altruistic motivation in dogs almost inevitably adulterates reward-shunning people to the point of resorting to violence or the threat of violence to get the job done. Very few trainers who sneer at positive reinforcement types utter statements like, "Well, it's just that I prefer pain, fear, and intimidation as motivators." They imply (or directly state) that their dogs "respect" them, perform "for them," or have a good "work ethic." Noble schmoble. I admit to having more respect for trainers who honestly acknowledge that they choose aversive motivators to train their dog than I do for trainers who threaten and hurt under the cloak that the only real motivator is their personal charm or the crafting of some sort of dog super patriot.

There's also an element of narcissism to limiting respect and admiration to the set of virtues that are (nearly) uniquely human. Evolution has crafted some pretty awe-inspiring strategies for making a living in the world, with our splendiferous brains calculating the whats and whys of other splendiferous brains around them being but one. Hell, we can do it recursively. "Do you think she assumes I'm firing him because of what he did to Frank?"

So, at the risk of sermonizing, here goes: Being kind, respectful, and generous and associating oneself with intrinsically good things does not cheapen or corrupt relationships. Your dog loving you and having fabulous associations to the wonderful things you do are not mutually exclusive. One won't trump the other. They egg each other on, truth be told. And being violent or threatening toward someone, in whatever guise, is not character-building. The fact that relationships can and often hang on in spite of regular delivery of pain, startle, and intimidation does not make coercion good. And everyone in the behavior modification field is well aware that it is absolutely possible to modify and control behavior—of adults, children, babies, dogs, cats, horses, birds, bunnies, and any animal you can see without a microscope—with pain, fear, startle, and the threat of these. The question is: is it okay?

Some years ago, Dr. Suzanne Hetts, an applied behaviorist in the Denver area, was engaged as an expert witness in a court case wherein a dog trainer had accidentally killed a dog while employing a correction-based training method (using it as directed, not "misusing" it). Under the municipal anti-cruelty statute, the case should have been a slam-dunk. But because the defendant called himself a dog trainer and could hold up books wherein the technique was described, he was acquitted, as he was considered to have been within "industry standards."

I am not so naïve as to think I can sell the average force-oriented trainer on just how frankly inhumane what they are doing is by describing an extreme example. "It's a far cry from" arguments will kick in like antibodies to protect their psyches. But, I bet I can mobilize people who care about animal welfare to stop turning a blind eye to what goes on in the name of dog training. What goes on in 2008 is eye-popping, and it goes on in the face of years (decades actually) of proof that force, pain, fear, startle, et al., are unnecessary, not to mention scores of treatises laying out exactly how to achieve the same end with no coercion or violence whatsoever. There is no longer any information shortage about training methods. Trainers vote with their feet, training the way they feel comfortable.

It used to be that you could raise your kid any way you wanted and that "interference" from outsiders was a breaching of sacrosanct family autonomy and—here comes the big buzz word— freedom. No more. Sooner or later, the way Western society is progressing, the use of metal chains and electric shock to train dogs will be illegal. I wonder who wants to be the last one to give it up.

Pavlov in Everyday Life

I used to be on a Flyball team that practiced every Thursday night. Some team members swore their dogs knew it was Flyball night long before being loaded into the car and taken to practice. In one case, an hour or so before the trip to class, a garbage truck reliably came grumbling through the neighborhood right outside

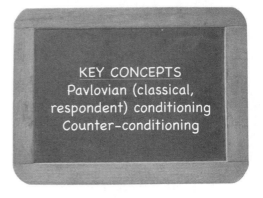

the family's house. Shortly after this, the dog would display excitement by barking, trembling, and racing around. This was well before any more obvious "we're going to Flyball practice" cues began. Another team dog would head to the door as soon as the owner changed into jeans and a sweatshirt after coming home from work, again, a good hour before departure.

There was a third dog who also started hanging around the front door eagerly between thirty and sixty minutes before leaving for practice. This one, however, had no identifiable tip-off that we could figure out. The likelihood was that the passage of time was the tip-off for this dog. Dogs, like many animals, are fantastically good at estimating time intervals. If there is any regularity to go on, dogs learn with startling accuracy the timing of important events to them: owners arriving home, daily trips to the dog park, meal times, nail-clipping day, and Flyball practice night.

These are all examples of classical conditioning, the form of learning whose details were worked out by Ivan Pavlov around the turn of the last century. Those same details have bored generations of psychology students in introductory classes, an obligatory rite of passage to sexier psych courses on fancy aspects of the mind. There's no doubt that classical conditioning is wildly out of fashion in psychology, but it's a goldmine for dog owners. It illuminates many of our "why does he…" questions and is a royal road to controlling—yes, controlling—our dogs' opinions of things.

Even in the hard-core dog behavior world, classical conditioning is usually muscled out of the way by its flashier cousin, operant conditioning. Operant conditioning is the science of reward and punishment and all the fascinating detail of exactly how dogs behave to get more of the former and less of the latter. Classical conditioning is the grim science of the inevitable. In classical conditioning dogs learn tip-offs to important events, and though they can't do anything to increase or decrease the likelihood of these events, they can prepare themselves: brace themselves if something rotten is coming up, and get a head start on, say, cheeriness or digestive juices if something fabulous or tasty is on the way.

I use the term "tip-off" deliberately. Teachers of classical conditioning often try to engage student intuition with the word "association." The dog forms "associations" between vet waiting rooms and vaccinations, between the upper pantry and cookies, and between hands reaching for his collar and being yelled at. A vital element needs underscoring in these examples: the predictive order of events. Vet waiting rooms come before vaccinations, the owner goes to the pantry before producing cookies, and the collar grab precedes the punishment. The order matters. It's just not good enough for one thing to happen "around the same time" of another thing. One has to reliably predict the other. Tip-offs to events that have already happened aren't very advantageous. No use bracing yourself for something that's already come and gone or, for that matter, is already here. The only tip-off worth learning is one that lets you know what is about to happen.

The Rules

So, the first rule of classical conditioning is to ensure the thing you're trying to condition the dog to love or hate comes first. If you want your dog to like Fed Ex deliveries more, go to the pantry and produce cookies after the Fed Ex man comes. Not before and not at the instant he arrives. After. Fed Ex deliveries thus gain predictive value. The order of events is an area where our intuitions can fail us. Partly this is an unfortunate by-product of the way classical conditioning is often taught to undergraduates—using the phrase "forming associations," which is not quite accurate enough. Remember: Pavlovian conditioning is more about anticipation, animals learning tip-offs to important events by virtue of their predictive value. Tip-offs aren't useful during or after, only before. The first event in a classical conditioning procedures says "here it comes…" and the second event is It.

The next rule for good conditioning is getting as close as you can to a one to one ratio of event one (delivery man) to event two (cookies). If the delivery man only predicts cookies half the time, conditioning will be weaker. If the non-cookie half happens when the owner is not home, the dog will learn this clause and thus feel warm and fuzzy and salivary when the delivery man comes and the owner is home, and much less so when the delivery man comes and the owner is not home. Dogs are very good at Specific Case.

The third rule for robust conditioning is narrowing the dog's focus to exactly what you want conditioned. Just as you feel smug that your dog has gone from territorial frenzy to wagging cookie anticipation, you discover the dog still hates (or is non-committal about) Fed Ex employees, but now loves people with clipboards! The real world is messier than psychology laboratories and dogs often selectively attend to—from our perspective—the wrong bits. To raise our chances of their attending to the right bits, a crafty trainer will break rule two for the wrong bits by proving to the dog in day-to-day life that clipboards predict nothing. As clipboards routinely appear before dog-dull activities such as watching TV or computing, the dog is more likely to go on uniformed strangers as the cookie tip-off when the Fed Ex man returns. So it's worth time thinking about whether there are any screamingly obvious things (to the dog) that might steal the thunder from your project. The usual suspects, competition-wise, are Big Stimuli—like smells—and elements in the training set-up that the dog has prior experience with—bait pouches, containers, the "I'm training you now" look, etc.

Finally, bear in mind that Murphy's Law dictates that all three of these rules for strong conditioning will align perfectly when we don't want conditioning at all. For example, dogs with separation anxiety usually start unraveling while the owner is preparing to leave for work. The dog trembles, pants, paces, or hides while the owner dons work clothes, packs a briefcase, and picks up keys. The reason for the dog's behavior is that the rules of conditioning have been dumbly followed: 1) the get-ready-for-work ritual comes before the owner's departure, giving it tip-off value; 2) the ritual is strongly correlated with being alone, giving it close to a one to one ratio; and 3) the ritual occurs while the owner is still home, resulting in the dog focusing on the right bit (the owner's activities) from a conditioning perspective, though of course the wrong bit from our perspective. Because such dogs feel anxious before the owner departs, separation anxiety treatment protocols must be broadened to incorporate desensitization to these learned tip-offs to aloneness.

Exploiting Pavlov

There are three ways to get classical conditioning to work for rather than against you. The first is to make a list of things you'd like to manufacture a favorable opinion about in your dog and start ensuring these things predict meals, cookies, walks, and play. For example, don't just brush your puppy; brush him briefly before every walk. Pack cookies (or, even better, beef jerky) on your walks and, every time your dog meets a child or hears a loud noise, provide a cookie afterwards. Rather than simply feeding your dog twice a day, grab his collar and then prepare and offer his dinner.

The second way to exploit Pavlovian principles is called "counter-conditioning." Let's say that rather than having no particular opinion about being brushed, your dog hates it. Adding a brushout before walks is not just conditioning any more: it's counter-acting an existing strong opinion. Counter-conditioning is often done in conjunction with desensitization, e.g., doing two or three light brush strokes before walks for a week, then five or six for a week, then five or six vigorous strokes for two weeks, all the way up to an entire (and happy) brushing in front of the walk.

Plain conditioning is usually easier than counter-conditioning: an ounce of prevention is worth a pound of cure. Puppies are thus opportunities. List everything you'd like your puppy to like as an adult and condition each one while he's still a puppy. Likewise, "first impressions" for adult dogs are also opportunities. Dogs are attentive—at least briefly—to new stuff. Capitalize on this. Imagine the dog asking, on first trips to the groomer, first car rides, and first collar grabs: "hmm, this is new—what does it mean?" Then answer the question: "it means cookies!" Indelible in many cases.

The final way of getting classical conditioning to work for rather than against you is the "don't lie" rule. If you're about to bathe your dog and your dog hates baths, it's relationship suicide to approach the unsuspecting victim saying "it's okay, it's ooookaaaaay" and then bathe him. Yes, you were able to easily catch him, but you also made your approach (or possibly "it's okay") a tip-off to bad news. If it's going to be bad news, signal bad news. "Bath time" said in a deadpan tone may send the dog running but, more importantly, you have protected yourself, your approach, and your soothing tone from unwanted conditioning.

It's also helpful to break things down into manageable chunks, to avoid elements in grooming that are likely to be intrinsically unpleasant. For instance, build just being in the tub up with some conditioning before doing the first bath. Do a few trials on the sound of the water. Do some on pretend (dry) "lathering." Separate foot restraint from the nail-clipping implement before clipping nails. Reeeeeally try hard to not hit the quick the first few times you actually trim. Likewise, do brush touches first and separately from restraint. Time invested in a new puppy can set her up for a lifetime of not just tolerating, but feeling happy and relaxed, during grooming.

Prompting and Fading

Dear Jean,

A friend of mine and I just got back from a clicker confer-ence and learned some great techniques. One thing that puzzled us was the stance many speakers took against lures in training. We were told over and over that lures would block true learning and impede our dogs' devel-oping greater intelligence and problem solving. We love the shaping techniques, but do we have to use them exclusively to avoid ruining our dogs in some way?

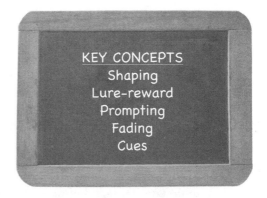

KEY CONCEPTS
Shaping
Lure-reward
Prompting
Fading
Cues

The pure shaping versus lure-reward debate has been going on for years with neither side offering up much in the way of blind em-pirical research to support their position that their way is "better," "faster," "more efficient," teaches dogs to "think," or grows "bigger brains." This hasn't shaken the most zealous in either camp from their biases however. And, like you, I've noticed the assault offense from the shaping crowd in the last year or two with some interest. It is frankly detrimental to see clicker training, which has so many merits, being associated with disdain for data, weak reasoning, and straw man arguments against the use of lures. It's unclear to me whether this is a vocal, visible faction of doctrinaire clicker funda-mentalists or a more widespread sentiment.

Let's define some terms before examining the merits of the arguments against the use of lures in training. A lure is an example of what behavior analysts call a prompt. A prompt is defined as an antecedent stimulus (something that comes before the behavior, as opposed to a consequence, which comes after the behavior) that is likely to elicit (achieve without any training) the desired response. Once the desired response occurs, it should be reinforced as usual. There are different kinds of prompts:

Physical prompts. These push or pull the animal into the behavior. In dog training they include pushing down on a dog's rear to make him sit, sweeping front legs out from under a dog to make him lie down, guiding with a leash, etc.

Lures. A lure is a non-physical way of steering an animal. In dog training, typical lures include moving a morsel of food held near a dog's nose to obtain sits, downs, stands, heeling, and other movements. Other commonly used lures are crouching, clapping, making high-pitched sounds, and retreating to prompt recalls.

Models. Modeling means providing an example for the subject to imitate. This kind of prompt is used in the training of some primate (notably humans) and bird species, but doesn't work in dog training as dogs are not good imitators.

Verbal prompts. Humans' ability to use language opens up a cornucopia of prompting options. For instance, when teaching manners to a child, an adult might say, "what do you say…" to prompt a child to say "thank you," or provide clues such as the first letter in a word to help someone guess a verbal response. Although sometimes trainers may feel they are using verbal prompts on their dogs to "remind" them of what to do in a given circumstance, they are more likely using cues as prompts.

Cues. Once a behavior has been trained and has a cue attached to it (e.g., the word "sit" reliably makes a dog sit), the cue can be used in the prompt position in order to establish a new cue. For example, in a (verbal cue) "sit" trained dog, to transfer control of the behavior to a context such as being let in from the yard, the verbal cue could be given after the dog presents himself at the door. Or, if the trainer would like to establish a finger signal to cue a trick, the finger signal would be given followed by the already learned verbal.

This last bit, about the unlearned leading to the learned, or to a prompt, is critically important but sometimes omitted by dog trainers. Although we are discussing operant conditioning—animals learning about the relationship between their behavior and its consequences—the relationship between a cue and a prompt is a classical relationship. The first stimulus, the new cue to be learned, is in the conditioned stimulus "slot" and the prompt, or known cue is in the second, unconditioned stimulus "slot." If the first event—new cue—reliably predicts the second event—prompt or already learned cue—classical conditioning will occur and the animal will start to anticipate the second event and deliver up the operant behavior before the second event. Trainers refer to this as the dog "jumping the prompt." It feels to the trainer as though the dog is cutting to the chase—performing the behavior ASAP in order to get to the reinforcement part. If you say "sit" to your hand-signal trained dog, wait a second and then deliver the hand signal, he will, over time, stop waiting for the signal and start sitting as soon as he hears the verbal "sit."

If cues and prompts are presented at the same time (or backwards—prompt first and then cue), the cue will not be learned. This is one of the straw man arguments I talked about earlier. Learning is not blocked or overshadowed by using prompts in training. Learning of new cues can be blocked or overshadowed by presenting new cues simultaneous to prompts or already learned cues, but this is an error only an extremely neophyte trainer would make when using a prompt. By analogy, no one would take seriously a contention that clicker training is useless when the arguer's version of "clicker training" is the presentation of treat first, then click, so the contention that food lures block or overshadow learning or cues, based on a rudimentary technical error should be similarly dismissed.

More often than simply waiting for classical conditioning to occur, trainers deliberately fade prompts. It is considered prudent practice to start fading as soon as the dog performs readily for the lure and to fade gradually. For example, after three or four times prompting a recall with a staccato, trilling sound, clapping hands and a crouch, the trainer might move to a semi-crouch for a few repetitions. If performance remains strong, every few repetitions she might reduce first the hand clapping, then drop the crouching altogether, then drop the hand clapping altogether, then reduce the vocal prompt in stages, culminating in a dog that comes enthusiastically for a bare verbal cue, "come!" Unstated here is that these performances for faded prompts are still being reinforced, i.e., some sort of intrinsically valuable event, such as a food treat, initiation of a walk or tug game, is provided after the dog comes. Failure to do so represents a problem of too-weakly conditioned behavior, not a problem with the prompt. Focusing on specific antecedent events, such as prompts, does not exempt a trainer from the consequence end of things. Once again, poor execution of basic training procedure is at the root, not the use of prompting.

As for problem solving ability in dogs, this term needs to be better defined, let alone researched, before anyone, including me and including anti-lure types, can make fair statements about it being reduced by the use of lures in training. It also bears mentioning that in the pet dog training arena, the development of "problem solving skills" in the dog may not always be a priority objective.

In other fields of applied behavior analysis, from work with the developmentally disabled to teaching gymnastics, the gold standard in installing new behavior is a pragmatic mix of both shaping and prompt-heavy training methods. The burden of proof thus lies with the "pure shaping" advocates to provide credible data supporting any drive to eliminate prompts from the dog training field.

Shaping

Dear Jean,

I have been shaping my Tibetan Terrier puppy, Brad, to do off leash heeling and it was going well, but then we got stuck. I'm not sure whether this is a good method to be using. I had no problem training him to make and maintain eye contact while walking by my side, but he drifts out of position if I make a turn and won't stay in position without lagging for more than ten seconds. Also, when I don't say "sit" on a halt, he stays standing almost all the time. I have been saying "sit" before I halt rather than waiting to see if he'll do it—is this right? When can we start proofing distractions and locations?

KEY CONCEPTS
Shaping
Successive approximation
Criteria
Rate of reinforcement
Parameters

I think you've chosen an excellent method and that you'll get a ton out of it! A behavior like heeling, which has multiple components and well-defined objectives lends itself particularly well to the technique of shaping by successive approximation. This is a technique whose rules have been well laid out by uber-trainers such as Bob Bailey or in books such as Karen Pryor's *Don't Shoot the Dog,* but that also can prove fiendishly difficult. I'd say the difficulties stem from two sources: 1) the all-too human tendency to break the rules, and 2) the necessity of keeping track of criteria. Those same components that allow ready break-down of heeling into nice, smooth criteria steps, can overwhelm a trainer who isn't either naturally well organized or keeps detailed training records. Let's look at the rules and how they apply to heeling.

Criteria and Rate of Reinforcement

It is well known and inherently obvious that criteria for reinforcement must be selected from among behaviors already being offered by the dog. For example, if Brad never executes a right turn closer than foot and a half from you, setting the right turn standard at less than one foot means the dog will never be reinforced. No properly functioning organism, including a dog, will play a game they never win. But if the standard is kept at what the dog is easily achieving, how does one make progress?

The optimal standard to set is one where the trainer never "loses" the dog (dog quits trying), but that maximizes incremental progress toward the final goal behavior. It's all about efficiency. Setting criteria too high results in frustration at best and constantly losing the dog at worst, necessitating having to get him back to the game with ultra-easy repetitions and a re-build to where you left off. Setting criteria too low results in wheel-spinning. The dog cranks out the same old behavior, often in a minimalist fashion, and progress is slow or non-existent.

So, a good place to start is knowing how long between reinforcers your dog can tolerate before he quits and always set your rate of reinforcement so that he never quits. There has been some convergence by systematic trainers on the idea of ten reinforcers per minute as a default rate for a green animal learning a new behavior. This comes to reinforcement every six seconds, which may be partial explanation for why your puppy is falling apart on a new behavior reinforced every ten seconds. The final goal is likely to contain a duration requirement of a minute or two, but this parameter will build more smoothly when Brad has a sturdier heel.

So a good trainer will determine criteria based on optimal rate of reinforcement. The question therefore is not "what behavior is the dog already offering," but "what behavior is the dog already offering at the rate of reinforcement I'm after." It helps to arrive at this call to think about parameters.

Parameter Juggling

Parameters are the different pieces that make up a criterion. For example, heeling has position, duration, eye contact (if desired), automatic sits and how well they are executed (i.e., how straight), take offs after sits, turns, pace changes, and the conditions and degree of distraction under which the dog must perform. At any given moment in heeling, each of these parameters will be at a certain level. And, remember, the key to good shaping is optimal rate of reinforcement, which means sample-driven criteria with clear articulation of what degree of difficulty of each parameter must be achieved for the dog to be reinforced. In a complex behavior such as heeling, this usually means keeping track of your parameters. Failing to do so easily results in what's called a "criteria pile-up," where the trainer inadvertently raises difficulty on more than one parameter at the same time.

Here's an example. Let's say you've got Brad to the point where he will heel in a straight line in a quiet location with perfect position and eye contact for a duration of eight seconds for five out of five practice trials. And let's say on your training agenda for this week is to get your sits automatic, get right and about turns up and running with correct position, and extend duration to fifteen seconds. When working your automatic sit parameter, if Brad's sits are automatic half the time without a verbal cue on straight-line heeling with reinforcement every eight seconds, and you do stretches of heeling that are eight seconds long and then halt, Brad will get reinforced approximately every sixteen seconds—for half the time when he sits automatically. You will lose him and possibly feel shortchanged as you're only demanding eight second stretches of heeling. What's missing is criteria that support an adequate rate of reinforcement, which for Brad at his current level is every eight seconds. To get the sits automatic, drop the duration requirement on the heeling. Heel him for four second bursts to maintain your every-eight-second rate. Once he's nailing the automatic sits every time, you can bring the duration back in. If you wanted to continue to use your verbal cue, when you halt, give him a second to sit. If he doesn't, say "sit" and don't reinforce—reinforce only the sits that didn't need a verbal cue. The sit cue comes after the halt so that halting predicts the learned cue. Brad's anticipation rate will go up and you can drop the verbal. And don't forget to keep the duration component at four seconds to avoid tanking your rate.

When you decide to work on duration, keep the heeling simple and build the time gradually. Don't add back any other features—turns, halts, etc.—until he can do long straight-aways. When you start migrating to distracting locations, drop all other requirements as you'll have much more competition for his behavior dollar.

This process of back-burnering other criteria parameters when raising level of difficulty on one usually requires keeping written training records for complex behaviors to avoid criteria pile-ups. When individual parameters are perfected, you can start combining toward your finished product.

Part of the reason shaping is so engrossing an activity for both trainer and dog is its complexity. Most dogs seem to relish the puzzle solving aspect. This is unsurprising when you think about it. Working for parsed out rations is ideal mental stimulation for a species whose ancestors not long ago had to solve problems—i.e., hunting and successfully scavenging—in order to eat. For train-ers, it can be a test of technical mettle to learn and apply the rules. What has always interested me most about shaping is how often the rules go out the window in the heat of training, especially if the trainer has an emotional investment in the dog being trained. This most often crops up when one is training one's own dog. So, when things do not go swimmingly during shaping, one of the first culprits to consider is whether the trainer is breaking one of those basic rules I described earlier. Have another skilled trainer observe your session and/or your training notes to see if they can lend ob-jective eyes to your adherence to the basics.

Timing

One fabulously well understood technical skill is the trainer's tim-ing. This is the latency (lag) between the dog's execution (often the start of his execution) of the desired response and the delivery of reinforcement—or the signaling of impending reinforcement—to the dog. Because dogs are not privy to human consensus that sitting is better than scratching or that watching is better than sniffing, and because dog behavior passes rapidly, it behooves the trainer to precisely reinforce desired responses rather than responses that happen one or more seconds later. Imagine playing a "you're getting warmer game" with someone who told you that you were getting warmer whenever you moved slightly away from the target location and then became frustrated at your apparent agenda to thwart their training efforts. Or sent you for a medical work-up to diagnose a presumed learning disability.

The gold medal timing upgrader is the clicker. It allows the trainer to mark behavior for reinforcement at a distance and with terrific precision. It divorces dogs from pocket-watching or monitoring flinches toward bait pouches, thus enabling them to move their bodies—including their sensory apparatus—more freely and never miss a click. While clickers do not solve training problems like low rate of reinforcement or poor criteria setting, they are powerful tools to improve timing.

Deliver a primary reinforcer after every click: the relationship between the click and the treat is a classical one. There are no intermittent schedules in classical conditioning, only weaker conditioning. Click only when you are going to deliver a primary reinforcer. So, if a dog is on a variable ratio one out of three for "down," the two out of three downs that are unreinforced receive neither a click nor a primary reinforcer. Clicks don't mean "correct behavior," they mean "here comes a primary reinforcer." Every time you click without treating you weaken the charge on the clicker. There is no good reason to do this. If you wish to distinguish wrong responses from correct responses that are part of an intermittent schedule, develop a system to differentiate these. For instance, mark wrong responses with a signal such as "not quite" or "wrong" and say nothing for correct responses that are to be unreinforced due to the schedule. Or say nothing on wrong responses and mark correct responses with "good one," which means "that is the response—enough of those and you will be reinforced."

Clickers don't automatically give you superb timing. Clicks are often late and occasionally early. If you find yourself in the same shaping ruts again and again, consider videotaping yourself to evaluate your timing, or training with a coach whose job it is to monitor timing. The maxim is: you don't get what you want, you get what you click.

Intermittent Schedule Use

Speaking of intermittent schedules, Bob Bailey has rather persuasively argued that they are over-rated and over-used in practical animal training. For those of us who were taught about resilience to extinction and the need to employ dense schedules (two-for and three-for each reinforcer) before upping criteria during shaping, his contention is somewhat heretical. A strong contingent agrees with him. I am among them for the following reasons:

1. In most practical pet training contexts, behavior hasn't plateaued out in frequency to the point where it would be advisable, by the book, to bring in a maintenance intermittent schedule. We bring in schedules, I think, partly in our eagerness to get more for less, and to kowtow to the pressure from those uncomfortable with providing food reinforcers. But this is poor technique and defeats part of the purpose in pet dog training, which is to provide a work-to-eat environmental enrichment regime.

2. When raising criteria during shaping, if the new criteria level is selected from among behaviors the dog is offering at a frequency that will support an adequate rate of reinforcement, applying an intermittent schedule to the existing criteria is not necessary. For example, a dog sits ten out of ten times at the end of a recall. The trainer would like to reinforce straighter sits as her next criteria. In the spectrum of sits already offered, she can select a narrower "band" of straightness that supports a rate of reinforcement tolerable to the dog. From the perspective of an outside observer it might appear to be an intermittent schedule for the plain sit or a continuous schedule for the straighter ones. Ditto from the perspective of the dog. It could "feel" like an intermittent schedule for the old criteria or continuous for the new regardless of what's in the trainer's mind. So, at best, it's moot. At worst, however, if the trainer elects to put the plain/old sits on an intermittent schedule before selecting the new straightness criteria, the following could happen. Let's say of the ten sits,

four are straight enough to be reinforced under the new criteria. In the continuous-for-the-new-criteria regime above, all would be reinforced. Under an intermittent schedule of, let's say 40%, any 40% of the old sits might be reinforced, which is less efficient. Even if the trainer "tries" to select the "best" sits, this is inferior to an articulated criterion that the trainer can spot every time it occurs. The key to this efficiency is twofold: One, have a shaping plan before commencing, to reduce the need to "scout on the fly" for next criteria levels. And two, shift criteria when the dog is fluent at the current one and offering the next level in your plan at a level that will support a rate of reinforcement that particular dog can tolerate.

One time where an intermittent schedule—i.e., partial extinction—can be exploited strategically is when there is a genuine lack of variability in the range of responses being offered. To break the stereotyped and overly efficient style in the dog, an intermittent schedule invites variability of response, as though the dog were asking, "hmm—I used to be reinforced for this all the time but now I'm not—I wonder what it is about the ones I am being reinforced for—if I could figure that out, I could be reinforced all the time again" and then experiments. Voila: variability from which to select new criteria. This is not a strategy to overuse. It works best when increased vigor or intensity of responding is desired. Responses can also extinguish altogether. If you find yourself resorting to partial extinction a lot, it's time to re-examine your basic technique. Most shaping projects on most dogs will not require this.

Exploiting Premack's Principle

Dear Jean,

We are trying to train our Aussie, Norman, to stop attacking stuff. He is obsessed with the vacuum cleaner, the broom, and, if you can believe it, the bed sheets. A few weeks ago he suddenly went crazy while I was making the bed. As soon as I moved the sheets he pounced on them gleefully.

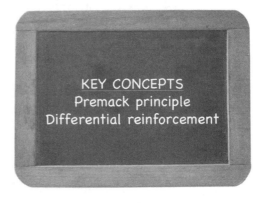

KEY CONCEPTS
Premack principle
Differential reinforcement

If I stayed still, he'd wait expectantly, kind of "go ahead, make my day" and then attack them if they moved. Norman graduated first in both his beginner and intermediate obedience classes and is well behaved at other times. He is sweet, affectionate, and has never shown any other sign of aggression. We walk him twice a day and, after this started, our instructor told us to increase his exercise so we made his evening walk longer and started playing ball with him in the backyard most days. He really loves fetch and it seems to tire him out, but he's still doing the Cujo thing with the vacuum. So we brought a private trainer out to the house and she suggested we put a training collar and leash on Norman in these situations and correct him by pulling sharply on the leash. After some reflection, we decided this just wasn't our cup of tea. On the other hand, he is not the slightest bit interested in our praise, patting, or treats at these times, so we feel stumped. Can we get him to stop doing this without resorting to hurting him?

There is a fiendishly clever and theoretically elegant solution to this type of problem. The catch is it's a very tricky orchestration job. Let's go through the theory first and then some nuts and bolts of the messy execution in your case.

David Premack is a psychologist who re-framed the concept of reinforcement as the opportunity to engage in a preferred response rather than the provision of a reinforcing thing, i.e. ,"eating is a reinforcing activity," rather than "food is a reinforcer." He also pointed out that the capacity of these behaviors to be reinforcing is relative, depending on the difference between the actual and preferred level of responding. What this means is that eating a turkey sandwich is likely to be extremely reinforcing if you haven't eaten for a couple of days, whereas eating a turkey sandwich minutes after over-eating on Thanksgiving is less likely to be a reinforcing event. Sleeping, taking a walk, or sitting in a chair watching TV are more likely to be reinforcing activities after eating a massive turkey dinner, but under other conditions might have lower value. And so on. More than one astute student has rightly pointed out to me that "it's all Premack" in dog training, meaning all reinforcement contingencies can be explained in Premacky terms.

Eyeballing an organism and guessing what the gold, silver, and bronze level activities are is impossible. You can, however, measure the relative frequencies of various behaviors when an animal has unrestricted access to engage in certain activities. The activities can then be ranked from high probability to low probability, depending on how much the animal does. The relative frequencies, as expected, will shift with shifting deprivation levels.

The most interesting part for us dog people is that the frequency of the lower probability behaviors can be boosted at any time by making the high probability behaviors contingent on them. Most kids wouldn't eat their broccoli (low probability behavior in the free operant baseline of a five year old), if they could cut directly to the ice cream (high probability behavior). So, as long as you know the order at any given time, you can manipulate frequencies. If you eat broccoli first, then you may eat ice cream.

Dog trainers have heard the maxim "turn the distraction into a reward." The sub-text of this is that what we label "distractions" in dog training are actually motivators that are trumping the motivators we wish to employ. From the dog's point of view, these are not "distractions" at all. As a matter of fact, to a dog that is trying to investigate the rear of another dog, the trainer (waving food or yanking on a leash) is the distraction!

Now for the messy application part. The objective with Norman is that he refrain from attacking your household goods (low probability behavior), in order to get to attack your household goods (high probability behavior). The first dicey bit is your willingness to grant the motivator, at least often enough to maintain the polite refraining. If you never, ever want him to do these things, even in short bursts at times you specify, then Premack's Principle can't be exploited. Granting access is often a prohibitive consideration in predation situations. Take squirrel chasing. Sometimes the squirrel gets a sufficient head start if the dog does a recall before being granted opportunity to chase, but sometimes chasing is unacceptable in any form to the owner and/or there are other safety considerations such as traffic, or animals being skunks and porcupines rather than squirrels.

If you think you might be willing to give him short, cued bursts of attacking the sheets and vacuum, then the next issue is engineering it so that he cannot directly access these activities unless he has first done some polite, waiting behavior. At first, I suggest that you require from him only a short pause, an impulse control droplet, in order to grant him an attack. Then, very gradually, crank it up until he must do impressive amounts of polite down-stay to get brief bursts of attack reward. Imagine, if you will, consuming five or six servings of broccoli in order to get a tablespoon of your favorite ice-cream.

So, how to get those early impulse control droplets so he can dope out the rules to the broccoli-ice-cream game? First, proof an impulse control behavior, e.g., down-stay, until it is very sturdy around normal distractions such as food dropped in front of him, etc. He was top of his obedience class, so this part may already be in place. The next step is to introduce the vacuum. Because the down-stay is likely to be null set around it, and Norman needs to be set up to succeed at this early on, I recommend mechanically preventing him from screwing up by harnessing or holding him. This is admittedly clunky but it gets the job done. Use as little mechanical restraint as possible, partly because this can be agitating around a prey-type stimulus and partly because we want to monitor for any droplets of self-imposed impulse control. This first session may require two people, one to vacuum or move bed sheets and one to restrain and monitor Norman. It helps the cause to do the least provocative vacuuming or sheet moving possible.

Proceed to put Norman in his down-stay. The designated vacuumer then does a bit of vacuuming. If he lunges, the vacuuming ceases and the trainer/restrainer stops him and re-commences the down-stay. Repeat. Once he holds his stay, even a little, praise enthusiastically and then say "okay, GET IT!" and let him have four or five seconds of gleeful play. Then, tell him "out" or "enough" and re-commence from the down-stay. Most dogs get worse immediately after they sample the reinforcer a couple of times—this is fine. Persevere. In a few more repetitions, most dogs begin more keenly holding their down-stays, rapt and waiting for the "okay, GET IT!" cue.

Once he's good at it, re-training for each problem scenario goes faster as the task is sufficiently similar. You can even use this same reinforcing activity to sharpen up other obedience commands.

Ringwise Dogs

Dear Jean,

I show my yellow Labrador, Beatrice, in obedience. She has her CDX and we started competing in Utility two months ago. Over the span I've been training her, I've noticed a gradual deterioration in her performance of basics such as heeling, speed, and enthusiasm in her retrieving of scent ar-

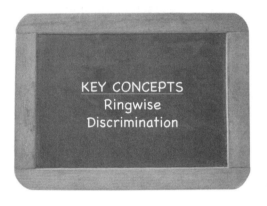

ticles and straight fronts. There are a lot of fronts in Utility! Here is the part that really bugs me. This deterioration appears only in the ring. In class and when we practice, she's near perfect. I've been told she's "ringwise," but what exactly does that mean? I've also been told I should do more matches. My handling is pretty good, according to my instructor, so I'm not sure I see the point of doing matches. Any ideas? Her heeling was actually sharper in Novice.

A ringwise dog has learned the difference between training and performance events. Although the exercises are the same for both and many of the context elements are the same—mats, jumps, scent articles, etc., there are enough differences to allow the dog to form a discrimination between the two. Once this discrimination is formed, the dog will respond to each depending on the learning contingencies each predict.

Why do animals have this discrimination capability? The answer is efficiency and, often, survival. Behavior must be orderly. Animals that employ "shotgun" approaches, one-size-fits-all responses featuring little or no match between behavior and context, are out-reproduced by animals whose repertoires include precise calculation regarding what to do when. I bet, for instance, that you don't try to walk straight lines and do square corners with precise footwork when you're on your way to work.

Animals also need to discriminate context to formulate motivational priorities when there is more than one option (i.e., pretty much all the time). If you're a prey species, for example, it would be maladaptive to dither between eating and anti-predator responses, such as flight, in the context of an approaching predator ("this is a particularly sweet patch of grass; I think I'll grab just a few more mouthfuls and…aaaaaaiiiiiiieeeeee…"). Animals with poor discrimination of context more often fail to contribute their genetic legacy to future generations. And so, good, adaptive motivational prioritizing evolved, and it depends utterly on context discrimination. Zebras don't try to drink the grass. Lions don't try to mate with trees (or zebras). And, in a learning situation, rather than acquiring a general case rule whenever they learn something, animals often code context cues to help them decide when to trot out which learned behavior. Which brings us to your girl.

Beatrice has learned that it pays—either to avoid punishment or obtain reinforcers, depending on your particular training tribe—to heel, sit, jump on cue, and do go-outs in the context of a training class or practice session. She has also learned that it does not pay, i.e., there are no behavior-consequence contingencies, to do these behaviors in a trial context. Trial contexts are quite particular. There's a high density of middle-aged women in polyester skirts and tennis shoes—a dead give-away for the fashion-conscious dog—clipboards, crowds, adrenalin, and human and dog stress hormones in the air. Ring barriers (curtains, baby-gates), stewards with nametags barking out numbers, and time spent waiting in crates complete the picture.

It's extremely important to note that there is no conscious agenda on Beatrice's part. In spite of deeply held trainer suspicions, dogs do not estimate the cost in entry fees and travel of an obedience trial and then craftily offer up lackluster performance as retribution for an abbreviated fetch game the previous week. A human might very well alter their behavior for these sorts of motives. Machinations based on theory-of-mind—e.g., I know you think I believe you were lying yesterday—are one of the strong suits of human cognition. Humans are prone to theory of mind misfires at dogs (who are, after all, Honorary Humans). These, combined with the human talent for reciprocal altruism—the evolutionary root of The Golden Rule—can make for a lot of wildly entertaining and oh-so human just-so stories about why dogs do what they do at obedience trials.

The bottom line is that, at an obedience trial, sitting straight, snappy retrieves, and sharp heeling don't result in the same consequences as they do in a training context. Motivational mileage can be obtained in the case of a dog that finds one or more of the tasks intrinsically reinforcing (e.g., Border Collies living to retrieve) and so not all dogs' performances deteriorate in the same way or even at all. When self-reinforcing features are absent, extrinsic motivators—or their glaring absence—will come to control performance.

It takes time for the dog's brain to dope out the rule—there are no rewards and/or punishments in the ring at obedience trials, but still/always rewards and/or punishments in training class—and behave efficiently. This accounts for the often-seen phenomenon of gradual deterioration over time, which is what you are reporting in Beatrice.

To reduce this effect, I have two suggestions. The first is to blur the distinction between the two. Add as many trial-type elements to your training picture as possible. The best way to do this is to go to matches, as you've been advised, provided you train at the match, i.e., provide rewards and/or punishments. For most dogs, matches are adequate trial simulators. Continue entering and training at matches—train just as you would in a training class—until performance has maxed out. This brings us to suggestion two, which is to avoid entering trials until the dog's performance is 1) as flawless as you can make it in matches, and 2) resilient to extinction. This means that you can, in training class or, more importantly, at a match, do the entire routine trial-style, from start to finish (with reinforcement at the very end, on exiting the ring, for instance), without rewards and/or punishers and without detectable flaws in performance.

Some trainers work around the no-feedback-in-the-ring problem by developing legal conditioned reinforcers that signal mid-routine that rewards will be supplied to the dog post-routine. A word or phrase, which has been conditioned over weeks and months to predict food, a favorite game or unabashed affection, can serve as a "you're on the right track, reward is coming soon" and help maintain performance.

Training Deaf Dogs

Dear Jean,

We recently acquired a deaf dog from Aussie rescue. Magic is a year old and housetrained, but doesn't seem to have even rudimentary obedience. We've had dogs before, but this is our first deaf dog. How do we train this guy?

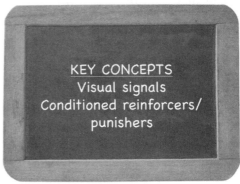

KEY CONCEPTS
Visual signals
Conditioned reinforcers/
punishers

A fine trainer and good friend of mine "specializes" in deaf dogs, offering, for instance, one free consult to anyone who rescues a deaf dog. I say "specialize" in quotations because he has made it abundantly clear to me that the principles of training a deaf dog are no different from those of training a dog who can hear. He is continually surprised, in fact, by how even experienced dog people go belly up when presented with a deaf dog, as though they must learn in a completely different way.

Deaf dogs, like normal dogs, learn from the immediate consequences of their actions. For example, a deaf dog will learn that coming to the owner in the dog park results 96% of the time in the leash being put on and the end of play. Being a properly functioning living organism, the dog learns to avoid the owner when called at the park. He can also learn that coming to the owner at the park results 85% of the time in a small treat and being sent back for more play, 10% of the time in nothing in particular, and 5% of the time in going home. In this case the dog is likely to have a strong recall. Dogs—including deaf dogs—do what works.

The difference with deaf dogs is that the communication system cannot depend on auditory signals. While any other sense can be exploited to set up a communication system, the two most often used are vision and touch.

The basic tools in any training system are:

- A conditioned reinforcer: a signal to tell the dog precisely when a behavior has worked, i.e., has earned him reinforcement such as a treat, game, door-opening service, etc.

- A conditioned punisher: a signal to tell the dog precisely when a behavior has made things worse for himself, i.e., has caused the termination of a game, withdrawal of a potential treat, or a time-out in the laundry room. I don't advocate physical punishment or coercion with dogs, but if this is your cup of tea, you can use yet another signal to communicate to the dog with the requisite timing that you're about to get violent.

- A set of cues for the behaviors you'll be training, such as "watch," sit, down, stay, etc.

Of these, the priorities are to teach Magic to watch you and to have a sterling recall. The most efficient first exercise combines watch with the establishment of a conditioned reinforcer. Before starting, decide what signal you're going to use to mark right responses: the "that exact behavior gets you a reward" signal. Most deaf dog trainers use a thumbs up gesture. Like all the visual cues, make sure it is clear and distinct from other hand movements you might use in everyday life. Get a supply of small, tasty treats and stand with Magic in a low distraction environment (somewhere in your house is fine). Stand still and wait, paying close attention. The instant Magic makes eye contact with you, even for a fleeting instant, give your thumbs up sign and then immediately deliver one treat. Then stand and wait for the next one. A sharp trainer will capture every instance of eye contact, which greatly accelerates learning. If you're crafty about catching every instance of eye contact and your timing is good, Magic will soon be quickly "recycling," which is trainer-speak for re-initiating eye contact immediately after being paid (treated) for the previous response. The behavior, which used to seem to occur by chance, now looks more deliberate. When Magic is recycling eye contact as fast as you can pay him for it, start delaying your thumbs up sign and payment for a second or two. The idea now is to gradually build duration of eye contact. Work your way up to five or ten seconds, only increasing the duration when he is recycling immediately.

The next step is to take your fledgling watch on the road. Re-teach the exercise in different rooms of your house, in the yard, in front of your house, with you at a bit of a distance, etc. Every slight variation may initially throw him for a loop, so be patient. This generalizing is well worth the effort if your goal is a nice, durable behavior. Once Magic is proficient in a variety of low distraction environments, practice around people and, finally, dogs. Outdoor coffee shops, in dog training classes, and in parks are excellent spots. Usually the standard has to be dropped back to that used in initial training (brief, fleeting watches) when increasing the distraction. Once the behavior is being recycled quickly, build back to your five or ten seconds.

Now it's time to add your "watch" cue so Magic knows when to do it. Decide what the cue will be. A common choice is a finger point to your eyes. Go back to inside the house. First, give the cue, then wait for the behavior and reinforce as usual. Repeat several times. Then, do not give the cue for a minute or so. During this no-cue period, ignore any eye contact from Magic. Then, give the cue and commence rewarding again. The nice strong behavior you've built should rebound nicely from the temporary wobbling it got when you stopped paying. Alternate these two conditions—no cue, no payment; if cue, payment for behavior—over and over until Magic gets the message: the behavior only works when the cue is on, like in the game Simon Says. This gives your cue value.

To teach a recall, first decide what the cue will be. Many trainers employ vibrating collars. A great web site, www.deafdogs.org, lists the available models, including the products' range, whether they are waterproof, lightweight, have a tone feature that would aid the handler in locating an AWOL dog and, importantly, whether the collar also can deliver shock. You don't need the shock feature. Electric shock—a sensation quite distinct from vibration—is not a desirable part of any animal's education. Just like in the previous exercise, train in a variety of low distraction environments before re-training around distractions. Increase the distance or move to a new location only when the behavior is performed with near 100% reliability. Start up close (a few feet away), using the following sequence:

1. vibrate the collar
2. after (not during) the vibration, encourage Magic to approach you (crouch down, run away, lure with food or even piggy-back on your thumbs-up signal)
3. as soon as he arrives, take Magic by the collar
4. give a generous reward—recalls are incredibly important, so don't be stingy
5. repeat

One of the first signs of proficiency will be Magic not waiting for the prompt (#2) but rather charging directly to you as soon as you vibrate the collar. When he's reliable and no longer waiting for prompts, commence your distance building and distraction-proofing efforts.

Managing Barrier Frustration

Dear Jean,

My Miniature Schnauzer, Max, is loving and clever. He loves to play with other dogs off leash and so we take him to a dog park most days for fun and exercise. I'd also like to be able to take him for more walks around our neighborhood, but herein lies the problem: Max ferociously

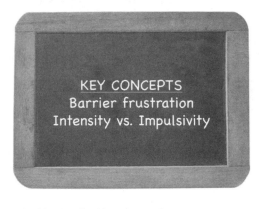

KEY CONCEPTS
Barrier frustration
Intensity vs. Impulsivity

barks, growls, and lunges at the end of his leash if he spots a dog, any dog (even a dog park buddy!). It is not only embarrassing, but concerning. Is he aggressive because he's closer to his own territory? Is it possible we have spoiled him with so much off leash play? Should we stop going to the dog park? How can we make Max more of a gentleman on leash?

Max's stellar off leash play history and wild man antics on leash strongly suggest that he is experiencing barrier frustration. Let's first gain some understanding of exactly what barrier frustration is and then get into how you might be able to dial it down.

We've all experienced frustration, a suite of emotions and behaviors in response to externally imposed limits. Psychologists studying frustration usually refer to concepts like the blocking of goal-directed behavior or the cessation of expected rewards. A car that suddenly won't start, a photocopier that jams when you're in a rush, and a spouse that changes the channel in the middle of a critical moment in your favorite TV show, all might elicit acute aggression in you.

Research on a wide variety of animals has shown again and again that frustration can elicit aggression. One psychologist in the 1930s went so far as to suggest that all aggression was frustration related! Nobody thinks this anymore, but there is good consensus these days that frustration can directly cause aggression and that the mechanism may be in the serotonin system in the brain. Medications that reduce impulsivity also mitigate aggression in response to frustration, suggesting a link between frustration-induced aggression and impulse control in general. It's also been found that within a species individuals will differ in the degree to which they respond to frustration with aggression. This certainly aligns with the observations of dog people. In what appear to be similarly frustrating situations, some dogs display signs of stress, but without aggression, some put on impressive aggressive displays, and some are utterly phlegmatic.

Dogs also seem to differ with regard to how impulsive they are, i.e., how hair-trigger they are in response to attractive environmental elements in general: smells, other dogs, people, ice cream on the sidewalk, critters, etc. Intensity and impulsivity are not the same thing. Intensity is partly a function of impulse control, but also of degree of motivation. A dog may be highly motivated by cats and so, in spite of otherwise great impulse control, lose it when he spots a cat. And a dog who is not necessarily off the charts motivationally may lack impulse control and so have zero lag between perceiving things and charging up to them.

Motivation can be cranked up with deprivation. Dogs and people become incredibly interesting to sociable dogs who are isolated for long periods. Chronic isolation situations can be very agitating. For example, long-term confinement to a backyard with a view of passers-by will often (and ironically) produce aggressive displays in what would otherwise be a friendly dog. Dogs with predispositions to guard when on the owner's property may also display at intruders, and so it's important in an individual case to ascertain whether a displaying dog is highly social and so primarily frustrated, or less social with strangers and therefore primarily guarding.

In Max's case, we're putting our money on frustration. My bet is he has some combination of strong motivation for dogs, possibly combined with impulsivity and, importantly, a tendency to respond to frustration with aggression. His behavior has nothing to do with being "spoiled." In fact, if you ceased your regular dog park outings, it's quite possible Max will get even worse on leash due to the more extreme dog deprivation. Barrier frustration is not at all a function of proximity to your home either. The worst cases of barrier frustration in fact are typically in kennels, where dogs are away from home (and far from spoilt). Kenneled dogs are, however, in a relatively static, barren environment, which increases their motivation to meet and investigate dogs and people, and over and over, they get to perceive (see, hear, smell) them, but can't fully and freely investigate. This frustrates many of the dogs and a percentage of these have the "respond to frustration with display" chip.

If you think about the lives of many dogs, there is an impressive amount of physical thwarting of strongly motivated behavior. Dog life is a continuous series of walls, fences, leashes, crates, and commands. Of course it's neither safe nor practical to allow free behavior all the time, but one way to reduce the load that might lead to barrier frustration in a susceptible dog is to mitigate these situations where possible. For example, if Max encounters a dog on his walk that he has demonstrated good off-leash relations with, try to pre-empt his displaying by hustling him over for an instant, motivation-deflating on-leash meet and greet on the street. Even better, do several in a row with that same dog, to practice manners. The first one, even if it ends up fraught with fireworks that will dissipate once Max has made contact, i.e., once the frustration is ended. The second one is likely to be a non-event: the "oh, you again" effect. This gives you a chance to praise and reward Max for doing exactly what you'd like more of in the future. Polite behavior on leash around other dogs. It helps to have a clearly defined behavior in mind to reward, such as "sit and watch me" or "walk by nicely" or even "approach dog without barking or growling." It also helps a great deal to use potent rewards: pack small, tasty food rewards for just such encounters. Praise and then feed good performances.

As Max gets more polished at this new game, you may start to get better results on even first tries with these familiar dogs. Continue to reward when he gets it right. If this becomes fluent you may start to see better behavior even around novel dogs. Consistently rewarding this will cause it to increase in frequency until, with some luck, it becomes his default.

Home Alone Training

Dear Jean,

My husband and I work full time. We have always wanted a dog. If we got one, the dog would be alone during the day from 8 a.m. to 4 or 5 p.m. Our neighbors, who also work full time, have one but the poor thing is in a kennel run pretty much 24/7. We really want a family pet. Is it realistic for us?

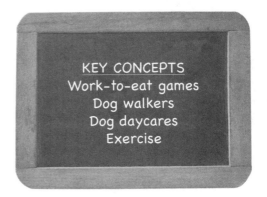

KEY CONCEPTS
Work-to-eat games
Dog walkers
Dog daycares
Exercise

It depends. You sound like good prospects insofar as you want to do it right. Lots of people work full time and give their dogs good lives. A common denominator is some attention paid to behavioral wellness. Dogs are social animals and eight or nine hours solo is tough from a mental health and behavior problems standpoint. But this can be mitigated. Let's look at how.

Dog Walkers

A fantabulous trend is the use of professional dog walkers, who break up the dog's day with a trip out, usually to a (safe) off-leash area with a pack of other agreeable dogs. Not only does this seriously reduce the likelihood of behavior problems stemming from under-stimulation (i.e., boredom), it gives the dog a mid-day potty break. While there is no question that a lot of dogs can be made to hang on to bladder and bowels for long hours, it is far from humane to do so. How'd you like to hang on way past what's comfortable on a daily basis?

If you go this route, check references and credentials. Ask the walker how she manages the dogs, how she deals with behavior problems, what first aid training she has had, and her plan in the case of injury or illness. Be sure you are comfortable with all of the above, and that she shows up when she says she's going to or sends a trusted assistant on days when she can't come.

Daycare

Doggie daycare has also become popular and a good daycare can add immense social stimulation and play opportunities for a suitable dog. The key phrases are "good daycare" and "suitable dog." A good daycare will have a low staff to dog ratio, such as one staff member per four or five dogs, takes care to put dogs in well thought-out groups (no hell-raisers with shrinking violets, no big with small), has some down/nap-time, screens dogs carefully for dog and people friendliness, and has impeccably clean premises. A suitable dog usually means a young dog who loves to play with other dogs.

Will Work for Food

If neither one of these is a fit for you, there are things you can do on your own to reduce the home alone dilemma. One is to throw away your food bowl and start using work-to-eat games instead. This is not inhumane—in fact, high-end zoos spend a lot of time developing enrichment strategies for their carnivore inmates, largely consisting of work-to-eat activities, and we would be well-served to take a page from their book.

For example, get a hold of enough Kong™ toys to hold your dog's breakfast. If your dog eats kibble, add baby food or canned food as a "matrix" to fill the gaps. Stuff the Kongs and put them in the freezer overnight. When you leave for work, hand the lot over to the dog. It will take him some time to obtain his food and he'll need a nap afterwards to recover. Yippee!!

If he empties the Kongs too quickly, increase the challenge: Stuff and freeze your Kongs, wrap each in a clean cloth and hide them around the house in different places every day. I once had a client who did this and put the wrapped Kongs in cheap plastic food storage containers or old margarine tubs. Very fulfilled little predator-scavenger she had.

If the first couple of days your dog leaves the Kongs untouched, don't fret and don't crack. No animal has ever starved himself to death in the presence of perfectly good food. If, however, this goes on for more than a couple of days, get him evaluated by a competent professional for separation anxiety, as anorexia when alone is a symptom.

It should go without saying that hard exercise is critical for dog mental health. Depending on your dog, the best option might be twenty minutes of fetch or Frisbee™ time at the local dog park or brisk walking. It really needs to be daily, so figure out what works and do it. If you opt for walkies, make sure it's long (thirty or more minutes) and that the dog gets to sniff stuff, to provide mental stimulation. Walks are seldom physically demanding for young dogs, but they can be very satisfying. My friend Janis was just today in fact marveling about a client consult she did where the dog—notably a terrier—didn't bark at the doorbell when she arrived (!) and was a happy and calm little thing (the clients were looking to improve his already quite stellar manners and behavioral health—trainers line up around the block for such clients!). Turns out he got six to nine miles of brisk walkies every day. I rest my case.

Training is also an under-rated "crossword puzzle for dogs." Even if you can't train your way out of a paper bag, provided you're not using pain, intimidation, or "corrections," your dog will likely enjoy the quality together time and, importantly, get mentally tired trying to figure out what the heck he's supposed to do to be rewarded. The process is the product here, which is why there's no need to agonize about how good you are at it. Get a copy of *Don't Shoot the Dog* by Karen Pryor, dream up some tricks or obedience behaviors, and get to it.

If you opt for do-it-yourself solutions, you are still left with the bladder-bowel issue. For this a dog door is the solution if you have a securely fenced yard. Otherwise, consider wee-wee pads or a turf box so your dog isn't miserably and desperately hanging on those final hours before you come home.

A great idea I've seen a few people come up with is neighborhood dog exchanges. If there's another family in the same boat as you nearby and your dogs are compatible (big "if" there), take turns having both dogs in the same house during workdays. This way the dogs get both a companion and a change of setting on alternating days.

Which brings us to the option of a second dog, or even a cat, for company. There are a lot of considerations here, the foremost being: does your dog like other dogs? I'm occasionally amazed at the lack of empathy in people who acquire a second dog in spite of the fact that the first one's life is made much worse, not least by the stress of having another dog around when she doesn't actually much like other dogs. Also, consider the double factor: double the food and gear, double the medical expenses, double the hair on everything, double the muddy feet, and so on. In the case of a cat, think very hard and possibly audition one to make sure your dog views this thing as a friend rather than prey item. And the cat needs to be a dog-lover, a tall order indeed.

Scratching the Rescue Itch

Like many dog people, I've been involved with animal shelters on and off throughout my career. And like many in the sheltering field, the satisfaction of saving and re-homing fantastic but unfortunate dogs in large quantities—be they diamonds in the flesh or diamonds in the rough—is why we do it. But also like many in the shelter-

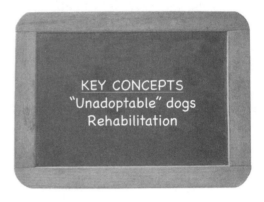

KEY CONCEPTS
"Unadoptable" dogs
Rehabilitation

ing field, I am often drawn—never by head, always by heart—to some dog whose luck is the worst of the worst. These are the kids whose intractable medical problems, ridiculously severe behavior problems, or some combination of these make them—by the standards of the agency in question—unadoptable. There's something about a dog having every conceivable genetic and environmental bad break that compels us Saver types to do our thing. Probably for the same reasons, I enjoy watching TV shows that depict dramatic re-models of dilapidated houses, and eye-popping hair, makeup and wardrobe makeovers of stressed out self-neglecting women. Fix fix fix!

For example, a friend and colleague, Kiska Icard, took on as a foster a teeny-tiny, rotten-toothed, occasionally ferocious dog named Violet whose age, overall ill health, and advanced heart disease gave her an estimated three months to live. Kiska—not without a full contingent of resident dogs already—took on the little thing for no rational reason and a year later carries her around to meetings in a dizzying variety of sweaters and jackets and cozy, plushy carriers.

Also about a year ago I happened to run into a fellow staffer, Mary, who mentioned that someone had dumped in our parking lot a neglected looking Chow. They had successfully cornered, poled, and gotten the dog over to Animal Control. She casually remarked that I might want to "go have a look." The wretched, matted, ill creature lay catatonic in the corner of her kennel. I don't know what it is about such utter hopelessness that propels one to act, but I ended up fostering her. I think that trying to help the hardest luck cases is like scratching an itch, an itch that seems not to get scratched by routine shelter work. In the service of this urge, I actually started up the world's smallest rescue, "Flip That Chow," where I make over the worst of the worst, one at a time. Now I recognize that I could use the time I spend on single extreme cases to help a larger number of dogs that are, uh, closer to prime time, but I participate in a fair amount of that in my day job and it doesn't deliver the same flavor of gratification that extreme makeovers do. So in my spare time I do a few of these.

Getting back to Buttercup the feral Chow, long story short, she ended up choosing her adopter by engaging with literally irresistible charm, John Buginas, who teaches with me at The Academy. John already had three dogs and was technically at maximum capacity. But she would have no other and we have since, with tongue in cheek, dubbed him The Chow Whisperer. The dog, now called Dax, seemingly unaware that she basically won the lottery, has blossomed into a virtual Chow Bombshell whose spectacular looks literally stop traffic. At the office we sometimes call her "Marilyn Monroe." John's wife has referred to Dax as a "walking piece of art." John has no regrets. It's as close as I've ever seen to a dog worshipping someone. Hearts fly out of her head when she sees John.

My latest (honorary Chow) flip is Gladys the Pekingese who flunked her body handling test on intake. Now the ramifications of an eight pound snorting thing that looks like it came from another planet trying to bite people are not up there with a fifty pound Chow being unkeen on humans, so right off the bat I figured I could phone this one in. And, as if to lull me further, Gladys sailed through the behavior modification process in a little over a quarter of the time a case like hers would normally take. Within a week she was handleable, groomable, eye-wipeable, ear-cleanable, foot-trimmable, tooth-scaleable, and so on. The home search began as did the inevitable impulse purchases of Little Beds, Little Glamour Collars and, notably, a stylish pink sweater. Fast forward to the other day. It is slightly chilly and damp. Gladys is in her sweater for the first time. She is fantastically cute and marketable. Pink is her color. We're coaching students on training plans in the Academy and John—that would be John the Chow Whisperer—goes to pick Gladys up and she growls. Can't be. All dogs (not just Chows) love John. And I fixed her. So we replicate it a few times. Growl, growl, growl. Debrief: there are a lot of other dogs milling around (possible minor factor), she is wearing her sweater for the first time (likely not a factor at all, but a new thing so must be considered) and, well, well, I hadn't proofed her newfound love of all things body handling with men (screaming 500 pound gorilla factor). A breathtakingly rookie move by yours truly.

So I have slunk back to the drawing board to tidy up my omission so she can get "perfect" back on her resume.

A Problem According to Whom? A Behavior Problems Primer and Overview

Dr. Ian Dunbar has famously pointed out that, although we call them behavior "problems," urinating on porous surfaces (like carpets), barking at intruders, and competing over resources are all normal dog behaviors. Problems arise when a dog's natural behavior or choice of outlet for it conflicts with our rules. And so the onus is on us to help our dogs better fit into our worlds.

KEY CONCEPTS
Management
Normalizing of normal behavior
Interrupt and re-direct
Systematic desensitization
Motivation/leverage

The key to prevention and treatment of most behavior problems is to manage your dog's environment in order to buy you time to teach him to employ "legal" outlets, i.e., ones you find acceptable. Think of it as cutting a deal with the dog that you can both live with. Twenty or thirty years ago, this approach would have been unthinkable for most trainers. The model then was that of a dictatorship, with the alpha-owner squashing all normal behavior in an effort to establish his or her dominance. But times change and the thinking of most dog trainers has changed. Part of the reason we love dogs is their very dogginess! And it's no longer seen as a slippery slope toward a coup to allow the dog expression of his natural behaviors.

For other behaviors, such as separation anxiety, noise phobias, and sharing high value resources such as food bowl or toys, the solution is to gradually acclimate the dog to these things as his genes did not prepare him well for them.

In all cases, it's much, much better to anticipate and prevent behavior problems than to undo them after they have become entrenched. Luckily, we know in advance what the likely problems will be so we can start off on the right foot with puppies or newly adopted adult dogs.

Let's look at the most garden-variety behavior problems first.

The Formula

For behavior problems like house-soiling, chewing furniture, and barking for attention, the recipe is:

1. Management. This means avoiding or breaking an undesired habit by controlling the environment so that more mistakes are physically impossible: you basically set the dog up to get it right every time! This usually means confinement. Under no circumstances should a puppy or untrained adult dog be free to cruise the house. Remember: it's always possible to relax rules later on when the dog has proven trustworthy, but it's very hard to go backward if you've set an early precedent of too much freedom.

Untrained dogs that are not confined will, quite predictably, eliminate when they get the urge, chew anything that seems a suitable chew toy (in other words, virtually all matter), and bark when they want something, such as attention, door-opening services, or a piece of your sandwich.

2. Train a legal outlet. Find an alternative behavior or a time or place for the behavior in question. The alternative must both be acceptable to the owner and meet the dog's need. Actively train this with lavish praise and food rewards. For example, if urinating on the carpet is wrong, what is right? Don't take it for granted when he eliminates outside. Be there right beside him to deliver a well-timed reward once he performs. If barking to be let out is wrong, what is right? Teach him that a patient down-stay gets your attention and those all-important opposable thumb-related services.

For behavior problems like chewing, digging, and other kinds of redecorating, part of the problem is that we provide free food to an animal that has a genetic legacy of having to hunt for a living. Under-stimulation, i.e., boredom, is a primary causative factor in many behavior problems. A full frontal assault is the best prevention: provide your dog with a wide variety of interesting chew toys; play fetch, tug, and hide and seek with his toys to burn off energy; provide regular dog-dog play; and, if he's really high-drive, get involved in a dog sport like Agility, Obedience or Flyball racing. Make him earn part of his daily food ration by unpacking stuffed Kong™ toys, hollow marrowbones, and by practicing obedience exercises or tricks.

3. Interrupt and redirect. When numbers 1 and 2 have been in place for a few weeks, reduce the confinement so the dog now has the choice of both the old (incorrect) and the new (correct) behaviors—if he attempts the old behavior, interrupt immediately at the start and redirect him to the new. For example, once the dog has demonstrated that he eliminates readily in the bathroom area of the yard and has been reinforced for a couple of weeks for doing so, give him some supervised freedom in the house and catch his first attempt to urinate inside. There's no need to be harsh—just interrupt him as he starts and hustle him outside to finish.

In some cases, supplying a (non-violent) penalty can help the cause, as in the following watchdog barking variation on the formula.

If your dog is inclined to go into orbit barking-wise when delivery people or visitors come, proceed as follows:

1. Manage. Try to arrange for a period of a couple of weeks where there won't be any real-life doorbell intruders while you work on your dog.

2. Ask yourself the key question: if this is wrong, what's right? If your dog loves people but simply barks too much, you can install a "quiet" on command cue by working on bark and quiet as a trick and then gradually increasing distraction. You can also

teach your dog an alternate behavior, such as down-stay on a mat (for mysterious reasons, many dogs can't lie down and bark at the same time!). Fetch maniacs can be taught that the doorbell is a cue to go find a particular toy.

When you have practiced and he is polished at the behavior, commence practicing with actual visitors. Be prepared to budget some attention the first few times toward reinforcing the new behavior in these real life situations.

3. Employ penalties—two minutes in the penalty box (bathroom or backroom away from the action) for infractions. For instance, if he holds his down-stay while the Fed-Ex man has you sign, he wins a piece of cheese. If he breaks his stay and/or barks after you've given him the down cue, he gets a two-minute penalty. If he barks in the penalty box, the penalty is extended until he is quiet for at least thirty seconds. Over time, he will learn that quiet is a strategy that works.

If your dog is actually uncomfortable with strangers ("takes a while to warm up" to visitors or is "reserved," "shy," or "protective"), the above watch-dog formula will not be enough. In this case, it is important to get at the underlying under-socialization. As prevention, socialize puppies extensively to as wide a variety of people and dogs as possible. You cannot overdo it. Expose them to plenty of places, experiences, sights, and sounds and make it all fun with praise, games, and treats. Find and attend a good puppy class.

If you missed the boat socializing your puppy, you'll have to do remedial work with your adolescent or adult. Whatever it is that your dog is spooky about must now become associated with his favorite things in the world, most notably food. If he doesn't like strangers, meals need to be fed bit by bit around strangers until he improves. It can take months to achieve noticeable gains with adult dogs so stick with it. I urge you to get competent professional help if your dog is not friendly toward strangers.

Certain individuals, breeds, and lines of dog are genetically more difficult to socialize. It takes greater effort, including formal behavior modification, to make them more comfortable with strangers.

Sometimes only minor gains can be made and their environment must be managed more carefully, both to avoid risk to strangers and stress to the dog. A stranger may be a kind, gentle person, but this is not relevant to a spooked dog.

Separation Anxiety

Dogs are highly social animals. Their genetic programming is to be in a pack with other individuals 24 hours a day, 7 days a week. They can learn to handle being alone for moderate periods of time but, in most cases, it doesn't come naturally. It's not surprising then that some dogs develop separation anxiety, a disorder which, in its severe form, can consist of panic attacks: urinating, defecating, frantically scratching and chewing at doorframes, barking, and crying whenever the dog is left alone.

Separation anxiety is often triggered by either a high contrast situation—months of the owner home all day followed by sudden eight hour absences—or some sort of life change—rehoming, a stay at a boarding kennel, a death of a key family member, or major change in routine. Not all dogs are susceptible—in fact most breeze through trigger events without developing a hint of the disorder.

Separation anxiety is both preventable and responds well to treatment. The treatment approach depends on whether the case is mild or severe. The first step is recognizing that dogs with separation anxiety are not misbehaving out of boredom, spite, or for fun. Some dogs with separation anxiety are fine when left alone in the car or fine when the owner leaves with slippers on to take out the garbage—they have learned the difference between "long absence" scenarios and "short absence" scenarios. Others are anxious in all contexts.

Puppies and newly adopted dogs are at higher risk to develop separation anxiety if they are smothered with constant attention their first few days home. It is much better to leave for brief periods frequently so the dog's early learning about departures is that they are no big deal and predict easy, tolerable lengths of absence: "whenever she leaves, she comes back." Soften the blow of your departures by providing extremely enticing stuffed toys for him to unpack. The first time you leave him for an extended period, tire him out with hard aerobic exercise ahead of time.

The "bored hunter" model is helpful here too. Give your dog both physical exercise and mental work to do. Not only does problem solving increase confidence and independence, it is mentally fatiguing and so increases the likelihood that your dog will rest quietly when he is left alone. Get him more focused on toys. When you play with him, incorporate toys. Hold chewies for him. Teach him to find a toy that you've hidden in the room and then celebrate his find with tug of war or fetch. Teach him his toys by name. Ask him to bring you one when you come home. Don't greet him until he's brought it. Then have a vigorous game of fetch. Teach him tricks, learn to "free shape" with a clicker, get him involved in a sport, and, if he's a playful sort, let him play regularly with other dogs. The more activities and toys are incorporated into his life, the less he will depend on human social contact as his sole stimulation.

Panic Attacks

If your dog is anxious to the point of panic attacks, he has severe separation anxiety and needs formal desensitization and/or medication.

In such cases, the informal interventions above will usually not help. What's needed is a formal program of systematic desensitization to change the dog's deeply ingrained emotional reaction to departure. The track record of systematic desensitization is excellent for resolving separation anxiety, however it is a huge amount of work for the dog's caregiver!

The key is to observe the dog for the first signs of anxiety during the owner's usual ritual prior to leaving the house. Most dogs with severe separation anxiety start becoming anxious before the owner leaves. They have learned the "picture" associated with imminent departure and begin panting, pacing, salivating, whining, or hiding. In fact, these symptoms of pre-departure anxiety are one of the ways separation anxiety can be distinguished from recreational chewing or behavior problems that result from dogs simply not understanding the rules or lacking outlets for their energy.

Once the kickoff point of the pre-departure anxiety is found, treatment begins by repeatedly commencing the ritual at this point, but not adding the subsequent steps or leaving, to teach the dog to relax in the presence of the cues that formerly triggered anxiety. Once the dog is relaxed, subsequent steps in the ritual leading up to departure and, finally, real absences are gradually introduced, always contingent on the dog's continued relaxation. The dog is then, over time, worked back up to normal length absences. Severe separation anxiety is a flag to get professional help.

Guarding of Food, Bones, and Toys

Possessiveness of food bowls, bones, toys, garbage, sleeping locations, etc., is natural dog behavior. Successfully defending resources from other pack members by threatening and biting is an adaptive trait, genetically selected for in wolves and feral dogs. It is an extremely undesirable behavior in a human environment, however. Luckily, most dogs can be taught to be relaxed and confident about relinquishing resources.

For example, to prevent food guarding, approach your puppy while he's eating and add a bonus to his dish—something much more palatable than his food. Approach from all angles and at different points in the meal and get others to do likewise. Hide the bonus and add it from your pocket or behind your back so it is not "previewed." Also practice removing the bowl while he's eating, adding the bonus, and then giving it back.

If your adult dog exhibits any of the following signs of guarding, get yourself into the hands of a competent trainer or behaviorist.

Signs of Guarding
- accelerated eating
- cessation of eating/"freezing up"
- glassy or hard eyes
- growling
- lip lifting
- snapping
- biting

Other Aggression Prevention Exercises

Teach puppies to bite softly by using time-out consequences for hard bites before forbidding all play-biting. Handle your puppy's body all over and make it fun with treats and praise. Find and enroll in a reward-method puppy kindergarten class that covers these exercises and allows free puppy play. Maintain socialization and comfort around resources and handling in adult dogs with regular practice. Maintain your dog's soft mouth by insisting he take treats gently and by carefully monitored and controlled physical games, such as tug. Allow your dog regular opportunities to socialize with other dogs.

Noise Sensitivity

Sound sensitivity manifests as fear of thunderstorms and/or sudden loud noises such as fireworks, gunshots, or cars back-firing. It is thought to have a strong genetic component. In some dogs it is evident from the time they are puppies. In others, there seems to be a gradual sensitization process, with full-blown sound shyness arriving around age two.

In certain cases, systematic desensitization can help using high-fidelity CD's. The dog is first exposed to the problematic sound at extremely low volume, low enough to not elicit any fear reaction whatsoever. A pleasant counter-stimulus is also helpful, such as giving the dog extremely high value treats after the sound has commenced. Then, very gradually, the volume is increased. This approach has a spottier record for thunderstorms in particular. For this reason, it's wise to supplement any attempts at desensitization between storms with management during storms.

Medication and Melatonin

Sedatives such as valium can be used to knock dogs out during storms. Valium is a better choice than a drug such as acepromazine. This latter agent will affect the dog physically but not provide any anti-anxiety properties. This can actually result in a more stressed dog—the original noise is still perceived, but now his motor skills are impaired.

Melatonin has received attention recently as an aid for dogs with thunder-phobia, other noise-related reactions, and other stressful situations. It is a hormone produced by the pineal gland in the brains of mammals. It is involved in circadian rhythms—those inner cycles that tell all mammals when to sleep and when to wake. In recent years, synthetic melatonin has been marketed for people as a "natural" aid to sleeping. Because published research is lacking, I can only report on the anecdotal claims.

The dose I've seen suggested for thunderstorm phobic dogs is: 3 mg for a 35-100 lb dog. Smaller dogs get 1.5 mg, and larger dogs may get 6 mg. The dose is given either at first evidence of thunderstorm or prophylactically before the owner leaves the house when thunderstorms are predicted. The dose may be repeated up to three times daily. The effects of melatonin on pregnant bitches are unknown so caution is advised.

One owner reported that his search and rescue dogs were successfully given melatonin to combat their fears of flying in turbo prop planes. It was the only treatment that allowed most of them to relax and yet let them perform their duties at the end of the flight.

Social Significance of Elimination

Male dogs may urinate on vertical surfaces, never fully emptying their bladders. Marking can extend to indoor locations. Neutering combined with training will solve the problem in most cases. The standard housetraining formula works perfectly well with markers. The catch is that marking is doubly motivated and there is no safe time envelope when the dog is "empty." Markers usually keep a reserve in their bladders. But the formula still works. Just be sure that management is very tight and vigilance greater in the interrupt and redirect phase of training. The next essay looks at marking in more detail.

Some dogs leak urine when excited or greeting. This submissive urination is an involuntary appeasement signal and should not be reprimanded as a housetraining mistake. To reduce submissive urination, keep greetings low key, avoiding both eye contact and looming over the dog. Establish a home-coming ritual such as fetching a toy or cookie-time in the kitchen to take the focus off gooey greetings. With these simple measures in place, most dogs' submissive urination improves as they mature.

Marking

Dear Jean,

Maynard is our Miniature Poodle. After I hosted a birthday party for him, he began marking in the house. He was neutered at age six months and is now two. He seemed to be having fun at the party, but perhaps felt threatened by the presence of other male dogs. I didn't see any of them lift their legs, but one might have when I wasn't supervising. Could this be why he started doing it? He is fully housetrained and still does all his business outdoors as usual. How do I get him to stop?

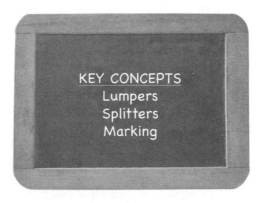

KEY CONCEPTS
Lumpers
Splitters
Marking

When it comes to behavior like marking, in the doggie behavior world, as in animal taxonomy, there are "lumpers" and "splitters." Splitters like diagnostic divisions and protocols that are precisely tailor-made to each one. Lumpers, whenever possible, throw as many of the splitters' divisions into one category, usually based on some less precise unifying feature.

Splitters view marking—the depositing of small amounts of urine in many places, usually vertical surfaces—as a completely different entity from garden variety housetraining. Super-splitters may make finer divisions still, such as: male vs. female urine marking, urine marking in males stemming from hormonal changes at developmental onset vs. male urine marking stemming from novel olfactory cues from other dogs and so on. A splitter would be verrrry interested, for instance, in doping out whether there were any urine deposits by those visiting dogs or not, details about Maynard's social maturational development, and quite possibly the visiting dogs' ages, reproductive status, and 2003 tax returns.

Lumpers are more likely to classify marking as, well, the dog peeing in the house. And then, accordingly, treat it as a housetraining problem with a regular housetraining protocol. In the case of urinating in the house, although there seem to be plenty of lumpers, I have not (thank heavens) come across any super-lumpers—people who might, for example, lump submissive urination, urinary tract infections, and geriatric incontinence in with housetraining/marking.

Some splitters acknowledge that their exhaustive diagnostic questioning can be overkill in the simple cases, but immediately point out that they will far less often miss the exotic stuff on first brush. And, some lumpers acknowledge that their cursory a-few-sizes-fit-all approach to diagnostics will result in missed exotica, but immediately point out that for most cases, they will be well into the final stages of training while the splitter will still be drawing blood and doing sleep architecture studies on the patient.

Most dog trainers and behaviorists are at neither extreme, though may lean a bit one way or the other. I am inclined to be a bit lumpy and so the advice which follows will help you not only get Maynard back on track (at least that is my lumpy contention), but—here's the fun part—also help you self-diagnose: are you a lumper or a splitter? If, as soon as you see what amounts to standard housetraining measures, you feel a welling up inside yourself of "No, no, no, idiot, he's perfectly housetrained, it's that he marks," you're leaning towards splitting. If not, you could be a more of a lumper.

Okay, on to Maynard. Yes, it is quite likely that his urination is motivated by something to do with the visiting dogs—the uncanny onset post-party at his age and after two years of perfection is the tip-off. But, although the motivation for urine marking is not identical to that in straight housetraining i.e., emptying of bladder vs. some olfactory or social trigger—the behavior is the same: the dog

is depositing urine in undesired locations. The dog in question has
the requisite spinal cord and so can be conditioned to deposit urine
only in desired locations, outdoors.

For two or three weeks, treat him as you would an untrained puppy. In fact, treat him as one of those untrained puppies for whom
you never have a safe, "empty" zone. Many puppies, once they
have performed both functions outside, can be trusted for a certain
amount of time inside, say half an hour. In Maynard's case there is
no safe zone. This is the one deviation from a standard housetraining procedure. Also, clean all the places where he has urinated with
an enzymatic, urine-neutralizing cleanser.

Crate or umbilical-cord (leash around your waist) Maynard when
he is indoors and not actively supervised. You may remember active
supervision from when he was a puppy. This is not the "I'm working on my computer and supervising the dog" kind, but the eyes-
on-dog-all-the-time kind. It really helps the housetraining cause
to have a two or three week period where the dog is prevented,
through diligent management and frequent enough outings, from
making even one mistake.

When he urinates outside where you want him to, reinforce him
with praise and, preferably, a small food treat. It must be completely unambiguous that he has done a glorious thing. In order to do
this in a timely manner, you have to accompany him outside for a
while. If he pees, then comes in and then is rewarded, it is too late.
The food must hit his mouth within a second or two of his com-
pleting his pee.

When this regimen has been in place for a few weeks, start loosen-
ing up the management when indoors. Stretch him for longer periods with eyes on him. If you see him wind up to mark, interrupt
him quickly and hustle him outside. Praise as usual. Sometimes the
first two parts of the regime—the management and habit-form-
ing—work like a charm and so no interrupts are necessary. But
often well-timed interruptions are vital, so it's really important to
be vigilant in this phase. If he succeeds in sneaking one or more in,
you're toast.

Most dogs, after a few interruptions, stop trying. Once you've had some weeks of vigilance but no attempts, you can start to slack off.

This procedure can drag on if there are compliance holes. If you kinda-sorta do it, it often won't work at all. Sloppy confinement, no reinforcement for correct behavior (the old "he knows, he doesn't need to be rewarded, blah blah blah" trap), or missing the first attempts in the interrupt phase can each derail the outcome.

Barking

Dear Jean,

I have a Pomeranian, Taz. He barks insanely when the doorbell rings or when the mailman delivers the mail. I read that the reason dogs bark at the mailman is that it works—the mailman comes, they bark and then the mailman leaves. From Taz's point of view, he drove away the

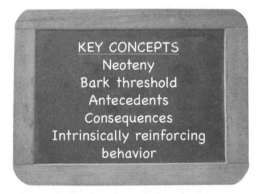

KEY CONCEPTS
Neoteny
Bark threshold
Antecedents
Consequences
Intrinsically reinforcing
behavior

mailman. But if that's so, then why does he still bark at visitors who ring the doorbell and I then let into the house?

Barking is considered a neotenous trait, which means it's an infantile or juvenile behavior that has been retained into adulthood. Dogs are directly descended from wolves and juvenile wolves bark whereas adult wolves seldom do. Dogs, by contrast, bark a great deal. Whether this was deliberately selected for during domestication or came along for the ride when other physical or behavioral traits were selected for is not known. There also seems to be significant differences among breeds and individuals with respect to how readily they bark, i.e., their bark threshold. Some are extremely phlegmatic, requiring a veritable marching band to prompt them to raise their head from a nap, whereas others, such as Taz, are hair-trigger, erupting into frenzy at the first hint of footfall from the mailman two doors down.

When it comes to modifying barking, it's useful to think about the antecedents and consequences of barking episodes. Antecedents are influential events that come before the behavior being analyzed. And consequences are events that immediately follow behavior. In the case of watchdog or territorial style barking, like you, I'm not sure I concur with the popular interpretation that it is driven by the consequence of seeming to make the mailman withdraw. Given the high proportion of watchdog barkers that bark regardless of whether the intruder withdraws, hangs out at the doorway, or enters, I'd venture that the behavior is primarily antecedent driven. If this is the case, then from a functional perspective, a more likely interpretation of watchdog barking is that it sounds an alarm or announces the presence of an intruder. I've often thought there is a dual purpose here, that of delivering an "intruder alert" to the owner as well as indicating to the intruder that he has been detected. It's not a stretch to see the usefulness of this trait, both during the time of domestication and today.

An antecedent control interpretation implies that the behavior is self-reinforcing—its very completion is its own reward. This is why the alterations in consequence—visitor departing, visitor staying, etc.—do not make much difference. The behavior has served its function if it has been triggered by the right antecedent. So, to modify it, it must either be brought under operant control—meaning insertion of the behavior into a consequence-driven sequence—or the antecedent must be addressed. Let's look at each of these strategies in turn.

To bring an antecedent driven, self-reinforcing activity under operant control, the behavior needs to be elicited and paid handsomely—at a level that will trump the intrinsic reinforcer—until the dog comes to expect payment for delivering the behavior. Jacinthe Bourchard, head trainer at Parc Safari Africain, a wild animal park near Montreal, Canada, makes the fabulous analogy about professional hockey players who, when they were kids, played strictly for the intrinsic reinforcement—the "joy" of the game. Players who then make it big in the professional leagues draw significant salaries and the behavior in many cases comes under this operant control—if the money then becomes insufficient, they demand more or even go on strike. Many other professionals report similar "corruption" of the original inherent pleasure they found in activities once they start earning money, acclaim, or other potent reinforcers for engaging in the activity. Amazingly, Bouchard has even witnessed this effect on strongly driven behaviors such as fixed action patterns in wild animals.

I have had success bringing barking under operant control by developing tight stimulus control over both barking and cessation of barking, by teaching bark-stop-bark-stop as a trick and then migrating back to the original watchdog context. But the above-described "professional" barking technique takes less legwork: rather than having to develop stimulus control first out of context, the trainer can train in vivo, simply delivering smorgasbords of food to the dog for barking when the doorbell rings. Eventually, these are withdrawn and the dog, in theory, goes on strike.

A classical counter-conditioning procedure could produce similar results. What appears to be behavior contingent smorgasbord is read as stimulus contingent smorgasbord to the dog and a competing anticipatory response to high end food is generated that then confounds the barking. From the trainer's perspective, it's a moot point—the easiest protocol to follow is to lavish heavy, heavy payoffs on the dog when he goes off in watchdog mode.

Another way to chip at watchdog barking is to turn the antecedent of a visitor, delivery person, or doorbell ring into a cue for the dog to engage in another behavior, one that is mutually exclusive to barking. For instance, a lot of watchdog barkers are terriers or herding dogs, who are, conveniently, often fetch maniacs. Before initiating any ball, toy fetch, or Frisbee™ games with these kids, ring the doorbell. Do not produce the toy and then ring the doorbell as that will result in the dog readily discriminating between intruder doorbells and fetch doorbells. Also, try to ring the doorbell without the dog seeing that it's you doing it. Arrange so that most doorbell rings result in the dog having to go to the back door, sit, and then go outside to play Frisbee or fetch. A minority of rings will inevitably result in you answering the door and there being a bona-fide visitor or delivery person, but even these can be followed up with a token game of fetch. As soon as the doorbell rings, prompt the dog, as usual, to wait at the backdoor post, let him out, answer the door, and then play briefly with the dog. This technique takes time to kick in, but is well worth it for industrial strength barkers.

If Taz is not much of a fetch addict, teach him to target and lie down in a specific spot. When he's proficient, add the doorbell—without a visitor—as a cue for the behavior. Then you can start using it in real situations. Most dogs can't bark as well in a down position, one of the mysteries of the universe. If Taz breaks his stay, cue and implement a time out, such as a minute or two in the purgatory of bathroom or laundry room. For busy-body dogs this is an effective and non-violent punishment that, combined with the alternative behavior training, can yield a nice result.

Oh Behave! Love and Mounting

Dear Jean,

My female dog mounts other dogs. Why does she do it? I assume she's dominating others. She'll be playing well with some dog and then suddenly she's mounting him or her! I find it obnoxious and so do many other owners. What's the best way to get her to stop doing it?

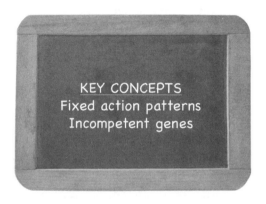

KEY CONCEPTS
Fixed action patterns
Incompetent genes

Ah, love. I'll tip my hand early and tell you the greatest likelihood is that mounting is a sexual behavior. In fact I think this one could stand some screaming from the rooftops: mounting is sex, mounting is sex, mounting is sex! That this is not obvious to any onlooker is actually pretty amazing.

Let's begin at the beginning. Fixed action patterns, or FAP's, are very important behaviors that are pre-installed in animals, kind of like bundled software that comes with your computer. They require no learning and are triggered by something in the environment. A classic example is a moving bit of string triggering a six week-old kitten to pounce. The pouncing sequence of movements is stereotyped across all cats. Another example is how a cat will turn sideways, arch his back, puff up and hiss. This is a self-defense FAP, again common to all cats and stereotyped.

Ethologists have coined the "Four F's" to refer to the four big categories of endeavor under which most FAP's fall. They are Fight, Flight, Feeding, and Reproduction. Animals that lack competency in their Four F's don't pass on their incompetent genes. One of the most interesting things about domestication is that occasional Four F incompetence might creep in—domesticated animals are no longer making a living in the world the same way as their wild forbearers so they can withstand dilution, drifting, or altogether dropping certain software programs without penalty. A cow without a well developed flight response is in much less danger than a deer. In some cases, breeding practices have deliberately magnified portions (think herding, pointing, and terrier stuff), softened them up, or greatly raised the triggering threshold for a FAP, such as in the case of Cavalier King Charles Spaniels who, for the most part, eschew fighting.

Cats are an interesting case as they retain most, if not all, their Four F FAP's. Because of this, there are many who consider them a semi-domesticated or even a non-domesticated species. Dogs, however, are all over the map, breed and individual-wise, with regard to Four F FAP retention. A given dog may or may not be very predatory (feeding), skittish and neo-phobic (flight), or highly competitive over resources (fight).

On to sex. At last. Reproductive behavior is, evolutionarily speaking, the biggest and most important of the four F's. Any animal that lacks super-duper strong courtship and reproductive FAP's doesn't pass on their ascetic genes. Genes are rather keen to get themselves passed on and so never neglect to install the "pass me on now" urge, action, and wow-was-that-ever-rewarding software in the animals they build. For the most part domestic animals retain reproduction FAP's, although technology like artificial insemination reduces the selection pressure even here.

Sexual behavior in animals has been studied a great deal. Female mounting is not at all unusual, especially during courtship. In one rat study I read, female mounting of what a girl rat considers a sluggish male was referred to as a "super-solicitational" behavior. Perhaps the rat equivalent of fishnets and a push-up bra.

In dogs, the courtship and reproduction sequence was studied in considerable detail by Frank Beach and Ian Dunbar (yes, the Dr. Dunbar) at the University of California at Berkeley.[2] A female who's ready to go might flirt with a male by mounting, clasping, and thrusting for a bit, then get off, run away and stop, hopefully with a super-solicited male in hot pursuit, not to mention oriented at the operative end of the female.

I don't mean to suggest that your dog is, uh, "loose," primarily because in play all manner of Four F FAP's are expressed in a giant jumble. In fact, the leading interpretation of why animals play in the first place is that they are rehearsing—perhaps de-bugging to stretch the software metaphor—key FAP's. Dog play consists primarily of chasing (feeding by the chaser, flight by the chasee), play-biting (fight and feeding) and wrestling, body-slamming, and pinning (fight), courtship, and copulatory behaviors such as paw-ing, mounting, clasping, and thrusting. These are punctuated by "meta-signals" such as play-bows, bouncy movements, and grinning play faces, which signal the playful intent of the F's they precede and follow. And note, all sexes might mount and be mounted by all other sexes: it's play. The chasee in a chase game isn't a real wilde-beest either.

So, when you say she's "playing well," I presume you mean she's bit-ing, chasing, slamming, and wrestling with other dogs. I am wholly fascinated by the sheer number of dog owners out there—you are in good company—that find these behaviors non-obnoxious, but consider sex play across the line or, amazingly, not about sex at all! Attend any dog park and you'll see owners continually and auto-matically defaulting to a non-sexual explanation for mounting, notably our old favorite, dominance. Now I'm no shrink, but unless dogs are way more into S&M than anybody has reckoned, when an animal mounts and thrusts, I think we need to rule out sex before entertaining other interpretations. In other words, when an animal does the grand-daddy of all FAP's during play, which is about FAP rehearsal, mightn't it be play sex, just like the play fighting, play predation, and play fleeing? Bottom line: Your kid is also playing

[2]Dunbar, Buehler, and Beach. "Developmental and activational effects of sex hormones on the attractiveness of dog urine." *Physiology and Behavior*, 1980 Feb;24(2):201-4

well when she mounts! In dog play generally, if a healthy dose of sex play wasn't present along with the other F's, it'd be a conspicuous absence requiring some fancy explaining.

I am not sure whether the abstemious streak in North American culture whirls us, like a centrifuge, away from the S word when we see copulatory behaviors during play or whether we're so dominance-obsessed, we co-opt nookie-nookie into some sort of power play. In any case, if you would like less of it, provide a non-violent consequence, such as a time out, whenever she does it. It could be two minutes outside the play area or, if you want to throw the book at her, march her back to the car and take her straight home. If, on the other hand, you think you might consider allowing her to do it during play, perform a consent test. If you suspect at any time that her partner may not be consenting, pull her off for a moment. Does the mountee grab this opportunity to get away? Does he or she hang out nearby? Or does he or she solicit play from your dog? This same consent test, by the way, works for pinning, wrestling, chasing, and other behaviors where there is any doubt about whether both dogs are enjoying the action.

The consent of both owners is also important. Although I have poked fun at some of the Puritanical motives that may be driving our 180 degree turn away from interpretations of mounting that involve sex, no owner at a dog park should be bullied by other owners, however well meaning, into allowing some activity with which they're uncomfortable, including mounting. If everyone passes the consent test, the dogs can proceed.

Car Whining

Dear Jean,

I own two Malinois, Nikita and Klaus, that I do obedi-ence, tracking, and Ringsport with. They are both outstand-ing working dogs. The problem is they drive me insane in the car, incessantly whining and yipping at this annoying pitch. I've tried crating them with covers over the crates to calm

KEY CONCEPTS
Pavlovian (classical, respondent) conditioning
Conditioned emotional response

them down, giving them chew toys to occupy them, spritzing them with water when they do it, praising them when they don't do it, pulling over and only starting again when they stop, and, in desperation, threaten-ing to kill them. Nothing has worked. And, whereas they used to do it only at the end of the trip to the park or training field, now they do it even when we're just running the occasional errand. I consider myself an excellent dog mom—we go to the park most days of the week and play fetch for nearly an hour. We also hike regularly. So, with all that exercise and with all those activities I mentioned, they couldn't possibly be under-stimulated! How can I get them to knock it off?

Car whining is among the most difficult behaviors to eradicate. The reason is that the type of car whining you describe is not driven by reinforcers or punishers, or by visual stimuli outside the car, which is why the standard measures you've used bounce off it. Nikita and Klaus were wide awake and taking copious notes in Intro Psych when Pavlovian conditioning was discussed.

A lot of dog behavior that is of interest to us is most readily modifiable by operant conditioning, the timely application of good and nasty consequences to increase and decrease its frequency. If a dog wants to go out in the yard, your act of opening the door is a reinforcing event. If barking makes you open it, barking is the reinforced behavior. If pawing the door makes it open, pawing is reinforced. And so on. If barking stops making the door open, it will eventually extinguish. The vast majority of dog people have some sense of this way of training.

Not all behavior, however, is most easily explained and understood in terms of its consequences. Some is best explained by the rules governing Pavlovian (or "Classical"), conditioning. For instance, take a sandwich instead of a door to the yard. If a dog barks and you give him some sandwich, barking goes up. So far so good. And, if you give him a sandwich when he stops barking, barking will go down. But, if the behavior is salivating instead of barking, you have a problem. No matter how expertly you communicate that the less he salivates, the better his chances of some sandwich, and the more he salivates the worse his chances get, salivation goes up. He ruins his own chances every time. This is because the anticipation of a piece of sandwich—involuntary salivation—trumps the operant refrain-from-salivating-for-sandwich contingency.

A lot of study has been devoted to what happens when operant and classical conditioning procedures interact.[3] When the interaction is a conflict, classical conditioning will tend to prevail. And so, back to Nikita and Klaus deafening you in the car.

Dogs are good at learning tip-offs to important events in their world. Leashes coming out of the closet tip them off that walkies are next, a set time of day tips them off that it's time for din-dins, and the sound of the garage door opener tips them off that mom is home. This ability to anticipate and thus prepare oneself for imminent events, gave animals that were able to do so an edge over animals that could not, and so classical conditioning evolved. The form the self-preparation takes varies, depending on what the

---

[3]A particularly good discussion of interactions between operant and respondent conditioning can be found in Schwarz, Wasserman and Robbins, *Psychology of Learning and Behavior 5th Edition* (WW Norton, 2002)

animal is preparing himself for. Salivation and gastric secretions are good preparation for food, and spikes of adrenalin and other stress hormones usually benefit animals who are about to fight or flee. Note that these anticipatory responses are involuntary.

While gastric, immune, and the plethora of other physiological responses that can be classically conditioned are fascinating stuff, what is most relevant to dog people are emotional responses. These are also involuntary. So, when a really, really fun and exciting thing has a reliable enough tip-off, a conditioned emotional response (CER) can develop.

High drive dogs, such as Malinois that can gleefully play fetch an hour a day and have leftover juice to excel in all those sports, are glorious CER fodder if some tip-off exists for all that orgiastic excitement. In your case, the tip-off is the car. So, the car whining is not driven by consequences or scenery, but an involuntary expression of emotional anticipation of the mind-blowing fun that ensues post-car ride.

Early on, Nikita and Klaus may have thought the car was just fine, or an ambiguous signal: sometimes just practice puppy car rides (if you took some), sometimes the vet (yuck!), and sometimes super exciting dog activities (SEDA). Over time, as you became a soccer mom—or rather a tracking-obedience-park-fetch-Ringsport-hiking mom—the car became a very reliable SEDA predictor.

In a simpler case, where the dog is frequently taken to a dog park and has a roaring good time, if whining develops it will initially commence toward the end of the journey there, say, in the parking lot. Then it bleeds backward to the street that leads to the parking lot, then to the turn onto the street that leads to the parking lot and so on. Eventually, the dog might start quivering with delight as soon as you load him up. If there is also a sufficiency of dull, boring car rides, and a few nasty ones for good measure, over time the dog will learn a finer discrimination. Load up can mean both, so isn't a good dog-park tip-off.

Clothing or gear can then come into play as discrimination aids. The best tip-off to whether any given ride is going to be to something great, middling, or hideous, however, might be the route. Leaving the driveway and early streets on the route are ambiguous, but a particular turn might be the tip-off that the park is the destination. In these cases, the dog's whining commences after the particular turn that spells park as destination. Failure to take that turn results in settling down or getting worried, depending on whether the dog has learned errands-only and bad news tip-offs. If a susceptible dog has too large a proportion of car rides to the fun place, car-whining can bleed backwards to the entire route.

One solution is to condition a confinement of the whining to the later parts of the trip by initiating more dull-o car rides that employ most of the route to the dog park, but then veer off at a critical juncture to endless boring errands. The dog will then learn that fork and gradually whine less prior to the dog-park-predicting turn. The whining gets compartmentalized.

Undoing whining in your dogs is a heftier challenge. They likely have multiple routes leading to all these varied fantastic things so have a general car ride CER. A regime of much more frequent super-boring car rides might help. If you can work out a way to compartmentalize the fun by developing a cue that means "good stuff is coming…," you might be able to kill or reduce it at other times. For instance, take a bunch of trips toward the fetch park, aborting at a certain point. At some point—hopefully sooner rather than later for your sake—the CER will start to extinguish. Once it's dialed down, alternate trips to the park with trips almost to the park that terminate in boring nothingness. On the real park trips, give a cue near the final turn: "wanna go to the PARK???" And then proceed to the fun fun fun. On the non-park trips, say nothing. The cue becomes a more reliable predictor than the car-ride. If it works, try a similar procedure for your other exciting destinations. By doing this you're exploiting the same laws of classical conditioning that got you into this boat in the first place.

Behavior Problems in Geriatric Dogs

Dear Jean,

Our Border Collie, Fly, is thirteen years old. Aside from some mild arthritis, she has no health problems. In the last few months, she's begun wandering around in the middle of the night, often waking us up. I don't think she needs to be let out as she keeps doing it even after we've just

let her out and she's pottied. During the day she snoozes more (probably tired from waking us up the night before) and wanders less, though she managed to wander behind the sofa and become trapped the other day. Is this attention seeking behavior or early signs of senility? She can play Frisbee™ and ball fetch as much as she did as a young dog so we know she's in good shape! Can our old dog be taught new tricks?

Old dogs are the dearest of souls and I have always considered it my honor and privilege to attend to their needs, especially after all they have given to us over the course of their lifetimes. You don't mention when Fly was last at the veterinarian. Even if she was in not too long ago, I recommend getting a thorough work-up done in light of these symptoms—things can progress fast at this age.

Changes in behavior in older dogs are not always signs of normal aging. Liver and kidney diseases, cancer, infections, and thyroid problems can all manifest as behavior problems. If these are ruled out, cognitive dysfunction is another possibility in your dog's case. Both her night-time restlessness and disorientation are flags for cognitive decline. The other symptoms are decreased ability to recognize familiar people and places, confusion or decreased awareness of surroundings, decreased activity, hearing loss, housetraining lapses, loss of appetite, decreases responsiveness to name or commands, and separation anxiety.

I can see both sides of the argument about whether to aggressively intervene or simply support dogs as they get older, but I do get alarmed when dogs are euthanized for treatable problems and miss out on quality months or years. House-soiling that is secondary to cognitive decline is an excellent case in point. This can often be improved with some knowledge and good veterinary intervention, and so it prompts me to urge people with older dogs to get them checked out and be given the latest and greatest in care.

In the case of geriatric onset separation anxiety, I know of many cases where standard departure desensitization procedures, which have an excellent track record for the disorder in younger dogs, failed to help. What did end up helping was addressing the dog's medical issues, which might include relief from arthritis pain, and dietary changes or medications to help with poor organ or endocrine function.

I urge you to not be lulled into complacency by Fly's zeal and stamina for Frisbee as her ultra-strong Border Collie drive to compulsively fetch can mask underlying ailments. In the film parody *Monty Python and the Holy Grail*, a game knight, after having both arms and both legs sliced off, exhorts his adversary that "it's only a flesh wound" and wants to keep fighting. I can imagine a legless Border Collie, seconds before succumbing to loss of blood, shrieking, "I'm fine, REALLY, c'mon, throw the Frisbee…" So get thee to thy veterinarian.

Alzheimer's?

The cognitive decline in older dogs has been dubbed "doggie Alzheimer's" and with good reason. In human Alzheimer's, the presence and quantity of beta amyloid plaques in the brains and blood vessels of victims are associated with the degree of decline in brain function. When geriatric dogs are so tested, a similar association is found. It is not known yet whether dogs suffer from reductions in key neurotransmitters such as dopamine and norepinephrine as has been found in human Alzheimer's patients. There is some suggestion that this may be based on the response of symptomatic dogs to a medication that inhibits the action of enzymes that metabolize dopamine.

The medication, selegiline HCl (Anipryl), was one of the early MAOI anti-depressant medications that has since been topped by newer generations of tri-cyclics and SSRI's for human depression and obsessive compulsive disorders. It has gained a second life, however, for treatment of diseases such as Alzheimer's in humans, which made it a logical choice to be tested for use in elderly dogs with Alzheimer-like symptoms. It fared relatively well and is now approved for use in dogs in both Canada and the U.S. Most veterinarians are acquainted with this medication and the diagnostic screening procedure put forward by its manufacturer. Dogs have been on Anipryl long-term without adverse effects. There are other drugs in the pipeline for human memory loss and Alzheimer's disease, however it may be many years before any of these trickle down to dogs.

It's not surprising that health care of older dogs is a hot topic among proponents of alternative and integrative medicine (which combines mainstream medical practice with nutrition, herbs, etc.). There may be changes in diet or supplements that would be in the can't-hurt-might-help category for Fly. For example, it has been suggested that certain B-vitamins, anti-oxidants, and even the herb Ginkgo Biloba might help preserve or even improve cognitive function. Free-radical reduction and scavenging are among the speculated mechanisms of Anipryl, so it's certainly plausible that anti-oxidants such as vitamin C, E, mixed carotenoids, alpha lipoic acid, Co-enzyme Q10, etc. could be beneficial. Omega-3 fatty acids, found in cold-water fish oils, are recommended to humans who wish to maximize brain function. Before implementing any herbs or supplements, be sure to run your plans past your veterinarian as interactions between medicines, herbs, and supplements are not always benign.

I am especially intrigued by evidence that exercising one's brain with new learning, problem-solving, and social interaction is a route to preserve brain function. This is something that could be also evaluated in dogs. Very often older dogs are sidelined, due to declines in performance levels, absence of behavior problems to motivate the owner to provide exercise and stimulation (i.e., they are more forgiving than younger dogs), and, in the case of multi-dog households, time and energy devoted to the performance activities of younger housemates. Perhaps problem-solving and learning activities—teaching old dogs new tricks—could be part of a comprehensive effort to keep their brains sharp into old age.

Understanding and Executing Time Outs for Dogs

Dear Jean,

I am muddled about the use of time outs—is it punishment and, if so, into what methodology camp do they fall?

KEY CONCEPTS
Negative punishment
Negative reinforcement
Inclusionary time out
Exclusionary time out

There are two kinds of consequence: reinforcement, which increases behavior; and punishment, which decreases behavior. Within each category there are two options, pain (the techie word for this is "aversives") and pleasure. It's very intuitive that pleasure is reinforcing and pain is punishing. What's less obvious is how pain enters into reinforcement and pleasure into punishment. When pain ends, it is (negatively) reinforcing—think relief from headaches, a warm house on an icy day, or switching off the blaring alarm you accidentally set off in your car. Aspirin taking, going inside, and putting the key in the car ignition are reinforced. When pleasure ends, it is (negatively) punishing—think Monday morning, removal of money through fines and taxes, or birders scaring away fantastically rare specimens by sneezing.

The continuum of training methods boils down to which of the above four types of consequence is used and how often. At one end of the spectrum are trainers who use primarily pain and startle and at the other trainers who use primarily rewards, or pleasure. In the middle are those who use combinations of starting and stopping pain and pleasure. Trainers who call their methods "pain free" or "without aversives" train by starting and stopping pleasurable things, which means they employ positive reinforcement and negative punishment. This is sometimes mislabeled as "operant," "no punishment," or "all positives." All consequences, including the most egregiously painful, are operant conditioning; negative punishment is, by definition, aversive-free and positive punishment is the kind of punishment where pain is involved.

Although the great wall dividing these approaches is whether pain is used or not, another interesting and more porous wall is that between trainers who use exclusively positive reinforcement (pleasure starting) and those who also use negative punishment (pleasure removal). There have recently been some claims floating around that time outs cause stress and side-effects comparable to those associated with aversives. Although I can find no research to support this, if such side effects actually do occur, there are a couple of possible mechanisms. One is separation anxiety. Negative punishment includes the removal of any reinforcing event or opportunity—food, a favorite game, or social access. When this last one is used in a dog that finds being alone not simply less reinforcing than being with someone, but actually distressing, the consequence bleeds over into positive punishment—i.e., aversives—territory.

The other possible explanation is frustration. When animals (including humans of course) experience abrupt cessation of things they like, they feel frustrated. The question is whether the frustration constitutes the same distress sensations that elicit fight or flight mechanisms. This seems implausible unless one considers cases where the reinforcer cessation is used with an animal already under chronic stress or where the criteria for gaining urgently needed reinforcers is deceptively unwinnable. Think Michael Douglas in the movie *Falling Down*, where every conceivable frustrating event of everyday life is thrown at his character in grim succession. In more mundane negative punishment scenarios, mild frustration can make the behavior appear worse temporarily. Puppies timed out for biting hard may briefly channel their frustration at being left alone into worse biting when the owner returns. Sometimes the opposite happens—the time out is a quiet time, and the dog seems more relaxed when the owner returns. Whether one particular time out elicits frustration or settles the dog down, however, its important thrust is as a consequence of previous behavior.

Time out is one of those techniques with an incredibly good track record for behaviors such as puppy biting or rude greeting, because owner contact is what the dog most wants at the time of the punishment. The catch is achieving all the elements of good execution. These are:

- Clear and consistent criteria and/or the use of a warning cue
- Timing
- Execution that avoids aversive elements, especially in sensitive dogs
- Compliance —the legwork issue
- The punishment must be punishing (!)

The dog will quickly learn what drives people away if the standard is unwavering. This means the owner must deliver time outs based on a certain degree of bite pressure, rather than based on how fed up the owner is or the owner's whim about what to tolerate today. A dog living with more than one person necessitates some estimating of what constitutes a hard enough bite for a time out. A warning cue makes the moving target of multiple standards much more navigable for the dog. This is a signal that means "you're on thin ice—the next bite like that one, or worse, and you'll be playing by yourself."

The punishment, once earned by a too-hard bite, must be delivered without delay. Otherwise, another behavior that occurs in the interim will be inadvertently punished. This is part of the rationale behind the owner yelping before giving time outs to puppies. The yelp marks the exact moment of transgression. Clicker aficionados will recognize this concept. The yelp (or other signal, such as "too bad for you") bridges between the crunch and the time out, a consequence that is difficult to deliver with razor sharp timing.

The delivery of the time out is ideally accomplished by leaving the puppy, rather than making the puppy leave you. The latter version is the one used to time out dogs for naughty behavior at the dog park or puppy class. There is potential fallout from collecting a dog to deliver a time out—any attendant leash or man-handling executed by angry or exasperated owners can take on an aversive edge, which invites side effects such as wariness of hands or approach in the dog. Luckily, with puppy biting, the owner can visit and exit the confinement area. This is the cleanest execution.

Which brings us to legwork. The owner must get up and step over the gate/leave the room, wait a minute or so and then return, and likely will have to do it again in short order. And again. And again. This is expensive behavior for people, especially given the absence of instant gratification—it doesn't work instantly. But to keep the standard clear and consistent, the owner must deliver the consequence every time. Non-compliance due to "legwork laziness" is a pet peeve of dog trainers. It only works if you do it.

Finally, the punishment—tautologically—must be punishing. For example, in the early education of humans there are two kinds of time outs, inclusionary and exclusionary. They are, respectively, time outs where the child remains in the social group, but is ignored and time outs where the child is removed from access to the social group. You'll occasionally see inclusionary time outs recommended for dogs: "cross your arms and ignore him" or "turn your back on him." In the case of a jumping-up dog who is most motivated by the owner's reaction, an inclusionary time out such as this could be punishing. In the case of a jumper who is reinforced by increased facial proximity, it very well might not be. A good rule of thumb for dogs is: if an inclusionary time out isn't working, try exclusionary. In fact, I usually recommend exclusionary time outs first for play biting or behavior that is elicited by a greeting context, i.e., the dog finds your presence the most motivating thing at that moment.

High Performance Dogs

Dear Jean,

My first dog just passed away at fifteen. She was a retriever mix and we did agility. I got really hooked on the sport, so for my next dog I am considering an Australian Shepherd, Border Collie, or Malinois. I've heard these dogs are high energy and I plan to keep mine very stimulated with agility and hard daily exercise. Any other behavior difficulties I need to know about?

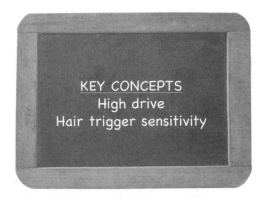

KEY CONCEPTS
High drive
Hair trigger sensitivity

Almost all breeds have behavior warts. Now, one person's warts are another person's virtues so what follows may very well warm your heart. And, a disclaimer: this is the opinion of one person. Talk to lots of people in these breeds to broaden your scope. And choose your breeder with care—sane, genetically clear stock, litter whelped, and raised in the kitchen rather than kennel, puppies handled, and socialized from day one, etc.

Serious agility people are drawn to high revving dogs such as the herding breeds on your short list. Herding dogs, like members of most groups, are not a perfectly homogenous lot, but there are notable behavior features common among them. One is "high drive," the thing that makes them excel at sports. High drive to dog trainers means a combination of ease-of-motivation—they are "driven" by moving objects and a compulsive desire to fetch and to tug, easily motivated with food or force—and perseverance or "work ethic." They focus well and will work longer and harder than many other breeds. This is one of the things that get them into trouble in pet homes.

Another tendency that can prove beyond the means of pet owners is their hair trigger sensitivity. The dogs you mention, and herding dogs generally, are spookier than the average dog. This might manifest as shyness with strangers, caution in new situations, sound sensitivity, or some combination of these. It could be that sensitivity is a good trait in a working herding dog. They have to be controllable in a quasi-predatory situation at great distances from their handler. It may also be, along with the drive, part of what makes them easy to train in contexts other than herding. The down side is a tendency toward neophobia—fear of novelty—and more ready acquisition of fears and anxieties along with occasional refractoriness to treatment once these are acquired.

In case I haven't already alienated readers with this somewhat bull-in-the-china-shop stereotyping, I'll now go further out on the opinion limb and say that herding dogs have a bigger than average talent for resource guarding, especially from other dogs. I think this goes part and parcel with the drive. Herding dogs value stuff. And some can be less tolerant than the average retriever about other dogs being around their stuff, or being around at all, especially when they're Busy. Which they very often are.

These qualities—high drive, high fearfulness, and high resource guarding—sometimes don't emerge until the dog hits social maturity at some time between ages one and three years. If this is a real phenomenon rather than just my idle musings, it means a fearless, non-guarding, and moderately drivey sheepdog at age ten months might morph into something more skittish, more possessive, and less tolerant of dogs by age three, without any particular errors or omissions in rearing. This is not to say that well-conceived and well-executed behavior modification can't attenuate or help prevent it. In fact, if I had to raise a herding dog tomorrow, I'd be super diligent in these areas with a view to prevention, and super-duper diligent in these areas if a problem were to arise in spite of my prevention campaign.

The worst case scenario is a dog strongly afflicted with all three traits. Such a dog has Aggression Redundancy, or three reasons to bite you and/or your dog: "you're a stranger, you moved irresistibly, and you went near my stuff/mum/park bench/grass." Treating these kids is gratifying—they love to do stuff, remember?—but requires breaking down the social shyness, movement sensitivity, and resource guarding components to make efficient progress.

I know slews of trainers with beautifully adjusted herders and also slews with herding dogs that, like fancy, imported sports cars, are in the shop a lot. To most in the latter group of trainers, it's a fair price to pay for the high performance.

Dogs and Cats

Dear Jean,

We are longtime cat owners about to add the first dog to our family. The rescue group says Clyde, who is a three year-old yellow Labrador, was tested with cats and found to be non-aggressive, very interested, and playful. Our current kitty, Dumpling, is ten years old and has never been around dogs. In spite of Clyde passing his test, we're still a bit worried. What's the worst case scenario? How should we handle the introductions?

> **KEY CONCEPTS**
> Species specific defense reactions
> Predation fixed action pattern

Kudos to your rescue group for checking Clyde out with cats. Very conscientious indeed. And equally astute of you to be careful. You are not out of the woods. "Interested and playful," while sounding nice on paper, might translate into some serious stress and headaches if things aren't properly handled.

Most adult cats who have not lived with dogs will react badly to a dog in their house. A dog, after all, is an active, (in this case) large, rude—by cat standards, animal. The correct terminology for your cat's likely reaction to Clyde is that she will emit "Species Specific Defense Reactions" (SSDR's). The non-technical term for this is "freaking out." It is critical in the early days and weeks that her initial hypothesis of Clyde being very, very bad news is not borne out by ensuing events.

The worst case scenario is this: Clyde gallops in with the restraint and discretion of a Labrador Retriever. Dumpling starts emitting SSDR's like mad. She puffs up, hisses, spits, slashes, and—here's the insidious part—peels away. From Clyde's perspective this is a Small Animal Running Away. The correct terminology for his probable next act is that Dumpling's flight will "release a predation Fixed Action Pattern" (FAP) in Clyde. The non-technical term for this is "chasing the cat." Which will freak Dumpling out more, giving her more reason to flee next time and ever more irresistible chase fodder for Clyde, and so on.

The way out of this cycle is habituation—for each, over time, to become slightly boring to the other. Pretty much everything in life gets old sooner or later, even cats to dogs and dogs to cats. The key is to control things enough early on so habituation kicks in before the above cycle can start ratcheting up. To do this, the earliest meetings need to have the following elements:

A. a well-controlled Clyde—behind a dog-proof gate and

B. a safe Dumpling who can absorb doses of Clyde at her own pace

Remember that even if Clyde doesn't put her in physical danger, it is enormously stressful for Dumpling to be confronted with a dog in the house. Dumpling needs space of her own that Clyde can't access. Clyde, as a newly adopted dog, will be gated in one or two rooms initially anyway (right?). This is ideal for Dumpling. Her food, water, litter box, and some comfy napping locations can be in the Clyde-free zone. This way she can approach the barrier when she feels like it. He will also get to see, hear, and smell her without risk of a fantastically exciting (for him) chasing incident.

Under no circumstances should you ever force them close together. Well meaning people have been known to firmly hold cats in their arms and march dogs up to them on leash. No amount of verbal encouragement ("it's oooookay") makes this okay. It is much, much better to give Dumpling 100% choice about the pace of getting to know each other.

As the days and weeks pass, Clyde will grow less fascinated with "Dumpling TV" and Dumpling will start to believe she is not going to die, or even be chased. You'll know you've reached this milestone when Clyde spends less and less time at the gate when Dumpling is in view and/or it is easy to break his focus when he is watching Dumpling. Dumpling will be hiding less and less as her curiosity gets the better of her and it becomes apparent Clyde can't get at her. When Clyde is out on walkies, she can hop over the gate and check out Clyde's stuff, hopping back to her sanctuary when he returns.

Once this juncture is reached, you may commence controlled meetings. Bring Clyde into Dumpling's space on leash with a bag of treats for both animals. Focus mostly on Clyde. The rule for him is: he does as he's told (i.e., down-stays for treats) or he has to go back behind the gate. If he was particularly eager to get at Dumpling in the earlier days, he may rev up again now. Stick to your guns. Go into Dumpling land and ask Clyde to down-stay (if you've never practiced this, spend a couple of sessions doing so before practicing around the cat). If he does, praise him and give him treats. If he breaks his stay, he is banished to his own territory. If you don't cave, he will learn quickly that it is very much to his advantage to hold his stay.

Coax Dumpling over with your voice and the treats. The idea is for her to develop a positive association to Clyde being closer, so make sure nothing bad happens. Something bad would be Clyde charging her. If you find it difficult to divide your attention between the two animals, attend to Clyde and sprinkle treats out for Dumpling. Use good treats, something she doesn't normally get. Clyde close by means treats.

If this goes badly, do the same thing, but with the animals on their respective sides of the gate. If it goes well, repeat it a few more times until Dumpling likes the exercise. She'll vote with her feet, so there'll be no doubt. The next step is to allow Clyde some movement still on leash. He no longer has to be in a down-stay, but he still mustn't come on strong to Dumpling. Praise and treat him for nice manners. If this goes well and Dumpling elects to hang around, you can remove the leash and, if that goes well, dispense with the gate. You may decide to continue to have one room where Dumpling can get away from Clyde. Many cat and dog owners maintain such a dog-free "safe room" for the cat even when there are apparently good relations.

Small Dog Syndrome

Dear Jean,

I don't know how to put this delicately, but are small dogs more neurotic? By that I mean are they more nervous, yappy, hard to housebreak and so get away with murder with their owners? And, if they are, is it in them or is it a result of the owners not treating them like dogs?

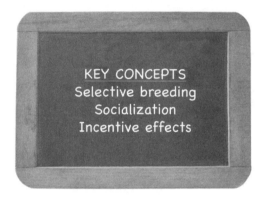

KEY CONCEPTS
Selective breeding
Socialization
Incentive effects

The only thing resembling research on the questions you ask is an opinion poll conducted by Benjamin and Lynette Hart some years ago on breeds and behavior. The Harts asked veterinarians, trainers, and groomers whether they thought certain breeds barked more, were more aggressive in certain situations, harder to housetrain, etc. Because it's an opinion poll (with all the baggage that comes with that approach) rather than objective research, it's difficult to gauge the accuracy. The good news is that the explosion of interest in dog genomics will likely lead to fabulous answers—and more sophisticated questions—in the coming years.

I'd venture that there is some consensus among my own group, dog trainers, that there are issues that crop up more often in small dogs. They are not dissimilar to some that you list: notably fearfulness, barking, and housetraining. Let's look at each of these for plausibility or evidence, and possible causes.

By nervousness you are probably referring to anxiety or fearfulness in social situations with strangers and/or other dogs. This could manifest as aggressive displays ("go away!") or avoidance ("okay, I'll go away!"). If small dogs do suffer from more than their share of social anxiety, the two obvious candidate explanations are genetics and socialization. The genetics question is best posed as: Does exerting selective breeding pressure to miniaturize an animal bring any fearfulness along for the ride? There are absolutely genetic mechanisms that could do such a thing so it's possible, but it's also far from proven. Socialization may be a more plausible explanation. Do small dogs get less socialization, on average, than larger dogs? The stakes are smaller—pardon the pun—if socialization is inadequate in a small dog and so perhaps there is a reduced incentive effect. There may also be some very understandable reticence on the part of small dog owners to expose their more physically fragile puppies to larger puppies and dogs.

There is a pervasive feeling that smaller dogs bark more but, again, this has never been looked at in a rigorous, scientific way. It would be easy to do: get a decent number of dogs representing size categories and count barks in the usual barking contexts. But it hasn't been done, so we're left to speculate again on possible causes for an effect that may not even exist. Genetics would be a possible explanation as would be the dog's day to day environment, primarily the owner variable. How does the owner respond to barking?

In the case of housetraining, I would be willing to bet that there is an incentive effect going on. Great Danes who still urinate in the house at age six months create massive, Def Con III incentives to buckle down and get the dog pottying outside, whereas Yorkies might elicit only sighing or eye-rolling. A lot of trainers feel that there's also a small-bladder/frequent-urination factor along with a more subtle squat that can make the little guys more challenging. Some trainers go so far as to indict certain breeds as being inherently, i.e., genetically, more difficult to housetrain. And, finally, owners of smaller dogs may be more ambivalent about whether to paper or housetrain the dog, and this can make for a moving target objective-wise, which might bog down training efforts.

There's an issue you didn't mention that I'm going to risk broaching, and that's owner or lap guarding. Some very otherwise charming little dogs can become ferocious looking when approached while in owner arms or on laps. This might be simply due to the fact that they can be in their owners' arms or on their laps, i.e., more medium and large dogs would do it too if they were ever attached to their owners in this fashion. Or it could be the incentive factor is lacking for both breeders to breed it out or owners to train it out. It's even possible some owners find it a bit flattering and so unconsciously reinforce it. For anyone with such a dog, the usual anti-resource guarding protocols work nicely as does the management technique of detaching the dog from oneself in potentially provocative contexts.

Tales From The Potty Training Trenches

"We reeeeeally need him to stop peeing inside." It started out completely routine. Melissa and Franco had called about recent housetraining accidents by their three year-old Lhasa, Mike. They clearly adored him, but said in no uncertain terms that this required amelioration. A few minutes into the history, Melissa idly leaned over

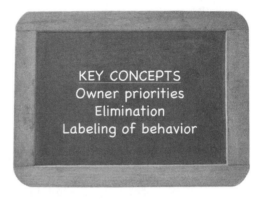

KEY CONCEPTS
Owner priorities
Elimination
Labeling of behavior

to scratch Mike on the head. Mike, lying next to his bully stick, growled and curled his lip. "Mel, wake up, he's on a bone here," Franco said, slightly annoyed. Melissa rolled her eyes, droning "I'm so senile." "He's done this before?" I politely inquired. "Oh yeah, he's a total freak around his bones and food." They chuckled nostalgically and showed me Mike bite scars. A minute into regaling me with a dazzling array of countless resource guarding war stories, Franco grew suddenly serious again. "Hey, listen—we don't check whether he goes when we let him out. I bet he's not even trying to pee. Do you think he might do something like that deliberately?"

Experiments have shown that nausea can be a stronger aversive than pain—animals sometimes work harder to avoid feeling icky, ill, or disgusted than they work to avoid shock. I started to roll this around in my head in relation to Melissa and Franco, but then snapped out of it and got back to work. They looked doubtfully at me when I floated the idea that the aggression was a) important, and b) modifiable. In fact, no amount of prompting and worse case scenario scare tactics got these people to re-prioritize or even acknowledge that their dog biting them to the tune of multitudinous punctures might be a Big Deal. "He just does that. We can totally work around it. He hasn't bitten us in—what—oh, two years. We keep him in the bedroom if people who don't know him come over." A pause. They beam at him. "It's kind of part of what makes him Mikey." They didn't say it, but I knew they wanted to add, "Can we pleeeeease get back to the peeing now."

I remember a call from a woman who urgently needed her elderly, obese terrier type dog, who resembled a bristly football, to stop peeing "everywhere." The dog turned out to have sleep incontinence and a happy ending veterinary referral, but not before I was treated to the sight of the football, sofa-ensconced with her owner, first gnawing on her sleeve: "nnnngaaaaaa" and then mounting her arm, with a full clasp and thrust. "Hmm. How do you feel about what she's doing right now?" "Oh, I'm just glad Dumpling still has enthusiasm for her activities."

People will live with all manner of stuff, but almost nobody will live with chronic house-soiling. Almost. I once did get a call for a young couple whose twenty-odd pound dog performed both functions several times a day on the wall to wall carpet all over their house. For four years. They shampooed the carpet every day. When I arrived, the tiny house, orderly and otherwise normal, reeked vaguely of feces and strongly of cleaning product. The dog was well groomed, fiercely loved, and they were mortified at the state of their home. They also seemed rusty at welcoming guests. By sheer luck, they had found out the week before the consult that something could be done. The Fed-Ex guy had gotten a whiff and said his own dog had been "fixed." I wonder if that moment for them was like suddenly remembering you had five hundred thousand dollars stuffed in your mattress. Kind of a combination of "this is too good to be true" and "you mean I've been clipping coupons for four years?"

A pretty common theme that crops up in housetraining is nomenclature. Labeling disagreements need to be put to bed before any actual counseling can take place. Take marking. "It's lovely to meet you and Thor. How can I be of assistance?" "He's perfectly house-trained, but he marks the furniture." Mirroring time. "So what I'm hearing is Thor urinates inside and you'd like him to do that only outside." "No no no, he's housetrained; he's MARKING." "By marking, do you mean he's peeing?" "Well of course." Most clients have the grace to not say "duh" at this point. "Okay, so the plan will be to get him to pee exclusively outside." Heavy sigh. "He already pees outside, we need him to stop MARKING." And so on. After a few of these, it occurred to me that I could leap-frog this agony altogether by leading with "Ahhhh, MARKING! Here's how we tame that baby." And then proceed to describe standard remedial housetraining. They do beautifully and everybody's happy.

Another obstacle to getting buy-in for the air-tight management and training regimes necessary to resolve most housetraining cases is the perfection of prior dogs. The vast majority of dogs kind of sort of housetrain themselves in spite of slightly half-assed efforts by their owners. Dog trainers are never presented with these house-training self-taughts. They are our invisible enemy. They are Lassie. And the mists of time improve them. A string of such dogs in the case of a particular owner sets up some mountainous expecta-tions, which then collide with any less easy to train dog that comes along subsequently. Most of these kids are not lemons, but they do require a by-the-book housetraining procedure. To an owner who has never had to do the by-the-book procedure, which requires a few weeks of genuine effort, it must feel like sounding out single syllable words for attorneys. "I have to do what? My last dog…"

The worst ever in the Dog Immediately Following Perfect Dog department was Mr. and Mrs. Burt, whose slightly PTSD-looking Cocker Spaniel, Glory, lay at their feet. To ensure razor-sharp tim-ing, Mr. Burt had done a stake-out in the kitchen during Glory's first weekend home. Whenever Glory would squat to eliminate, Mr. Burt would thunder "NOOOOOOOOO!!!!!" and whisk him out to the yard by the scruff of the neck. Glory, rather wisely, ceased eliminating around the Burts. He would wait, stalk still, in the yard, Mr. or Mrs. Burt on stand-by. From Glory's perspective they must have seemed like Dirty Harry looming over him, cocked and ready: "Go ahead—make my day…" He never found out it would have been scritchies and a cookie had he dared try on the grass. Then, as soon as he was alone, which only happened in the house, he finally relieved himself. In safety. Dog trainers affectionately call this reverse-housetraining.

What was shaping up to be trickier than average went into the flames when Mrs. Burt declared, frostily, "our last dog, Snowpuff, never made a mistake after the first correction. She lived to please us." Then, catastrophe. Not only had Snowpuff been a house-training savant, her back-story included bark-deterring bad guys attempting to break and enter. If they had laid out a pinned-under-tractor fantasy scenario I couldn't have been more discouraged. I tried the sympathy card. "Wow. That's sure a tough act to follow." Their eyes got all glittery. "Well, she's gone now, so we hope Glory will turn out to have redeeming qualities of his own." Ah. This might work.

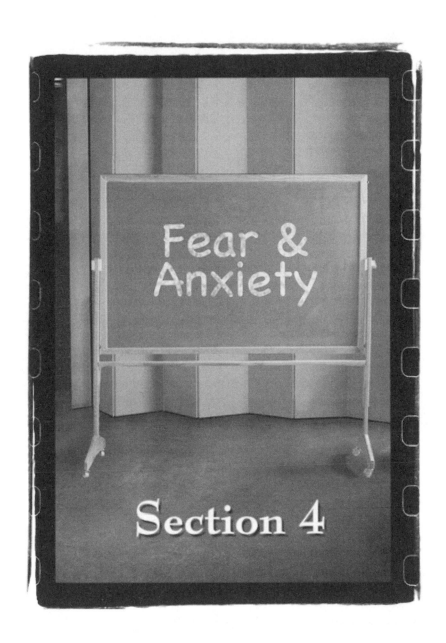

Fear & Anxiety

Section 4

Better Safe Than Sorry: Fear

Dear Jean,

I teach obedience classes. I encounter some owners of shy dogs that tell me their dog is a rescue and was formerly abused. If I ask for details, they sometimes can't supply any because they don't know anything about the dog's previous owner, which means the abuse is not actually docu-

KEY CONCEPTS
Behavioral determinism/
causality
Self-defense
Selection pressure
Classical conditioning

mented. Aside from the challenge of getting these people to move on from the "he's abused so we can't practice the exercise…" excuse, I find myself skeptical that so many dogs have been so badly abused. Aren't some dogs just shy?

If you are asking whether I think that behavior is without cause, then I would say no, I don't believe that behavior just "is." There are always determinants, even when we don't know what they are. If, on the other hand, what you mean is, "Are most or all shy dogs formerly abused?" then I think you are really onto something. I have observed, as you have, the tendency of people to invoke abuse as an explanation for shy or fearful behavior in dogs. It could be that people find it reinforcing to have taken on a hard-luck case. One need only scan the pop TV fare, replete with tragedy and against-the-odds comebacks, to know that humans are drawn to stories of the overcoming (or not) of egregious adversity.

Some of these dogs may have had abuse histories, but in reality, outright abuse is far from necessary to produce fearful behavior. Fear is incredibly easy to come by. The reason is that, in nature, when it comes to self-defense—the reason there is fear in the first place—the cost of a false positive far outweighs the cost of a false negative. What this means is that animals who err on the side of being too skittish out-survive and out-reproduce animals who err on the side of being too relaxed.

For example, let's imagine that you and I are two animals making a living in the world. You are the more skittish animal and I am the more relaxed. There will be times when an innocuous stimulus—something harmless—spooks you. There is a cost to these false positives. You wasted energy. You made yourself conspicuous while spooking. You might have hurt your leg running away. It might have been a food source you ran from. And so on. Now let's look at me, Ms. mellow animal, and what happens when I get it wrong, a false negative. There will be times when a truly dangerous stimulus fails to spook me. I'm toast as are all my theoretical descendents bearing my laid back genes. Ultimate cost. And so there is huge selective pressure on the evolution of fear. As it happens, there are different possible pathways for fear to use to get its job done.

What are the pathways? There are five. The first is genetics. There is ample evidence—in rodents, dogs, and humans, among others—that a predisposition to be fearful can be inherited. A well known experiment was performed on dogs by Murphree in the 1970s.[4] Commencing with normal Pointers, he bred the most fearful to the most fearful each generation, along with a normal control strain. After only a few generations, marked and seemingly refractory fear appeared in spite of normal rearing. It's important to note here that there is not one "fear gene," but rather a variety of genes that affect the endocrine system's physiology including neurotransmitter production, receptors, and re-uptake. Murphree clearly tapped into one or more of these.

[4]Murphree, OD. "Inheritance of human aversion and inactivity in two strains of the Pointer dog." *Biological Psychiatry* 7, 23–29 (1973) See also Newton and Lucas. "Differential heart-rate responses to person in nervous and normal pointer dogs." *Behavioral Genetics* 12-4, (1982)

The second way to get a fearful animal is via its prenatal environment, i.e., stress during pregnancy. In rodents it has been shown that stressing the pregnant female results in adult offspring with decreased stress resilience. The mechanism is the impairment of an important negative feedback mechanism in the offspring's hypothalamic-pituitary-adrenal (HPA) axis. This results in the adult animal having difficulty "coming down" once spooked.

The third fear avenue is maternal behavior. An experiment was done on dogs wherein two bitches, one genetically fearful and one genetically normal, were bred and then their litters swapped at birth. Predictably, the genetically fearful puppies reared by the normal dam were fearful but, interestingly, the genetically normal puppies reared by the genetically fearful dam were also more fearful than cross-fostered controls (ruling out the mom switch per se as a confounding variable). The mechanism couldn't have been genetics. So, was it the dam's milk? Some sort of social learning? Is it simply stressful being around a fearful mom? No one yet knows for sure.

Next in the fear production parade is classical conditioning. Dogs are not born fearing veterinary waiting rooms or the sight of nail clippers coming out of the tack box. They learn which things in their environment predict other, intrinsically scary things.

Finally, fear can be the result of impoverished early environment. It has been really well established that if you raise puppies through their socialization period, i.e., up to age twelve weeks or so, without human contact, they will be profoundly shy of humans. It has been further shown that a little intervention—some regular handling during this period for instance—greatly attenuates the effect. There is even some suggestion that enriched handling—i.e., mild (operative word mild here—a little is good, but a lot is definitely not better) daily stress for neonates—may increase stress resilience as adults. Where agreement disintegrates, however, is on the question of whether, once a puppy has been made shy by impoverished early environment, he can be turned around a little, a lot, or at all by subsequent intervention. Indeed, there is not much agreement about whether a fearful dog of any variety can be significantly improved. And, if it can, when and how can it—what individual case variables matter, what technique(s) work, and what is the time frame? Answers to such questions would assist prognosis estimates and treatment efficiency.

There is impressive agreement that fear is a much tougher nut to crack than most behavior problems. Even those, such as myself, who advocate that fear can often be greatly improved, emphasize that it is usually a much slower haul than installing manners, obedience, or resolving house-soiling. There is also pretty good agreement that diligent prevention—careful selection of breeding stock, socialization of young puppies, etc.—far outpaces treatment of an existing problem as a better option.

One of the difficulties with fear is its seemingly spontaneous worsening, sometimes as a function of social maturity, but other times due to its irksome property of generalizing, all by itself, to a broader range of stimuli than the original problem. For example, a dog that is fearful of large men with hats may erode to be fearful of large men without hats, then all men, then some women.

A sure take home message is that under no circumstances should one breed a fearful bitch, especially a suspected genetically fearful one. In this latter case, the puppies get blasted three ways. They get it via their mom's genes, they get it if their easier-to-stress mom is stressed during her pregnancy, and they get reared by a fearful dam.

Compulsive Disorders in Dogs

Dear Jean,

My husband and I have the most gorgeous fawn Great Dane, Muffin. Well, she WAS the most gorgeous Great Dane until she started licking her front legs six months ago. At first we thought she had some sort of seasonal allergy and that it would go away, but not only has it persisted but

> KEY CONCEPTS
> Compulsive disorders
> Conflicting motivation
> Redirected and
> displacement behaviors

it's gotten much worse. She has hideous sores on both legs and won't stop licking. We were going to take her for allergy testing, but our neighbor just suggested Muffin had obsessive compulsive disorder. Is this a physical or a mental problem? Have we made Muffin neurotic?

It sounds like Muffin has acral lick dermatitis, or ALD. The question of whether her problem is a physical or mental one is complicated. What kicks off ALD is often completely different from what ends up maintaining the problem. A classic case gets up and running when the dog has some physical condition such as a skin allergy or fungal infection, ringworm, scabies, demodex, nerve inflammation, arthritis, or even local tumors. Then, even if the primary physical problem fades or is resolved, the licking carries on. At this point the problem is considered a compulsive disorder (it's not known whether dogs have obsessive thoughts, so it's just called "compulsive disorder" in dogs rather than obsessive-compulsive disorder).

Compulsive disorders can be the end result of dogs trying to cope with frustration and conflicting motivation. In the frustration department, consider the life of many dogs: a fairly steady stream of not being able to access things they see behind fences and beyond the end of their leashes. Conflict might look like a dog who is simultaneously curious and afraid of the same thing. Another example is a dog who is sometimes greeted and sometimes punished by his owner in similar situations, such as when the owner arrives home or approaches. The dog feels a simultaneous urge to greet and avoid, which, if you think about it, can be crazy-making.

The acute feeling of frustration or conflict might result in a re-directed or displaced behavior. Dog trainers will tell you about getting redirected bites when grabbing the collar of a dog who is highly motivated to fight. The trainer is not the real target, but is unloaded on because she is handy and in the way. Displaced behavior, by contrast, is seemingly irrelevant to the context in which it occurs. The dog is conflicted so neither approaches nor avoids, but chases his tail instead. If the frustration or conflicts are chronic enough, the behavior becomes more entrenched and at a certain frequency gets dubbed a compulsive disorder. Once it's at this stage, it'll happen whenever the dog feels stressed or is bored and, in the most severe cases, virtually all the time the dog is not otherwise occupied.

Aside from acral lick dermatitis, also known as lick granulomas, compulsive disorders include (imaginary) fly-catching, flank sucking, whirling in place and tail-chasing, pacing, chasing shadows or imaginary objects, staring into space, excessive drinking, and self-mutilation.

Which particular behavior a given dog ends up with is thought to be at least partly genetically predisposed. For instance, breed over-representations include flank sucking in Dobermans, fly-catching in Miniature Schnauzers, and whirling in Bull Terriers. Lick granulomas pop up more often in Dobies, German Shepherds, and Danes, such as Muffin. Another potential determination of a dog's particular "choice" of compulsive disorder has to do with whether the original kick-off stressor was a repeated conflict or due primarily to the particular frustration of extremely low stimulation, i.e., boredom. Dogs who experience chronic conflict tend toward the high energy disorders such as tail-chasing or "popping" (jumping up and down in place) and then, once the disorder is entrenched, proceed to engage in their compulsion whenever they get amped up. Self-directors—like Muffin—might commence due to one of the physical causes described earlier, or conflict, and then carry on at times of low stimulation.

Another thing that can maintain ALD in particular is a vicious cycle of endorphin addiction. Once the dog has created a significant sore, the body releases its natural painkillers. If the dog ceases licking, the endorphins are not produced and the dog literally experiences withdrawal. So, the dog licks to keep the sore alive in order to produce the endorphins.

Before doing anything else, get Muffin to your vet for a thorough physical exam, bloodwork, urine, and a dermatology work-up. Depending on the outcome of these, s/he may want further diagnostics.

If the ball is passed to the behavior court, you should increase exercise and mental stimulation. Depending on Muffin's exercise tolerance—check with the vet on this—commence a daily bout of hard aerobic exercise. Perhaps more importantly, Muffin needs a Job to do. If there are courses in your area, enroll in something like a tricks class, musical freestyle, or advanced obedience. It doesn't matter if Muffin is a huge talent at the activity: the process is the product. We want Muffin's mind challenged.

An important caveat: be sure the course is taught using a punishment-free method. Regardless of what your personal philosophy is of dog training and regardless of any proposed merits of training dogs with correction collars, in the case of compulsive disorder resolution, removing punishments from the dog's life is a cornerstone of treatment. If there are no courses in your area, get a book on clicker training and learn to free-shape behavior. Karen Pryor's *Don't Shoot the Dog* is excellent.

It would also be a good idea to invest in chewies and puzzle toys—stuffed Kongs™ and activity balls where Muffin must roll them around in order to extract part of her meal ration. There's even a new device out that dispenses stuffed Kongs at pre-programmed intervals so Muffin can get unstuffing projects throughout the day when she's alone.

Teach and reinforce a behavior that is incompatible with forepaw licking. A good example would be fetching and chewing on a specific bone or resting her head on a cushion at times when she might lick. This is another place where clicker expertise might come in handy.

You and your husband must bone up on ways to communicate with Muffin in a consistent manner, specifically to avoid any sometimes-punish-sometimes-not conflicts that may occur. A well-run training course will teach you how to do this. Once again, be sure to screen carefully to be sure the course employs strictly reprimand and punishment-free techniques.

Consult with your veterinarian on a potential course of anti-obsessional medication. The tri-cyclic anti-depressant clomipramine (Clomicalm) and some drugs in the selective serotonin reuptake inhibitor class, such as fluoxetine (Prozac) and fluvoxamine (Luvox), have track records at working well in conjunction with the behavior modification measures listed above. In the case of ALD, hydrocodone, the narcotic agent found in Vicodin, has proved helpful in certain cases. Aside from providing pain relief, it has been speculated that an exogenous opiate source interrupts the vicious endorphin cycle. Using similar logic, opiate antagonists pre-empt the endorphin pay-off and render the behavior unreinforcing. This therapy is usually considered a last resort.

Understanding Psychotropic Medications for Dogs

Dear Jean,

Our Shar Pei, Angus, suffered for years from separation anxiety and, to our amazement and delight, was just successfully treated with a combination of training and an anti-depressant drug! It was a lot of work but we can finally leave him alone. I admit to being fascinated by the parallel of Angus and many people I know all being on Prozac! How do these drugs do what they do?

KEY CONCEPTS
Neurotransmitters
Serotonin
Melatonin

Medications such as fluoxetine (Prozac), amitriptyline (Elavil), and clomipramine (Clomicalm), achieve their effects by altering chemical messengers in the dog's brain. Neurons, the brain's specialized cells, are not in direct contact with each other. In order for the electrical signal from one to continue to the next, a chemical signal is transmitted across the tiny gap, called the synapse, between neurons. The chemical messengers are molecules called neurotransmitters. These molecules play a very important role in regulating our moods and controlling functions such as appetite and sleep, as well as emotions such as anxiety. Inside the terminal of each neuron are little pouches called vessicles that store each neuron's supply of neurotransmitters.

When an electrical signal travels along the neuron and reaches the terminal, it signals the vessicle to release some or all of its supply of a certain neurotransmitter. The neurotransmitter swims through the fluid in the synapse in a fraction of a second and contacts the neighboring neuron's receptors. There are many types of receptors. Like pieces of a jigsaw puzzle, each kind of receptor has a unique shape that allows only certain types of molecules to bind with it. A serotonin molecule will only bind with a serotonin receptor for instance. A dopamine molecule will only bind with a dopamine receptor. Once binding occurs, the neurotransmitter completes a circuit, stimulating an electrical current to flow along that neuron's axon, triggering the release of more neurotransmitters.

Once the neurotransmitter molecule has delivered its message, it detaches from the receptor. At this point, a number of things can happen. The neurotransmitter can keep floating around the synapse until it attaches to another receptor and triggers another signal. It can float back to its original terminal, where it will be sucked back up into a vessicle. This is known as re-uptake. Or, it can come in contact with another type of protein molecule called an enzyme, which will break it down to make it easier for the body to metabolize it.

This system is complex and a number of things can go wrong. The supply of a certain neurotransmitter stored in a vessicle may be too high or too low. The pump that re-absorbs the neurotransmitter during re-uptake may be defective, causing too few molecules to be re-absorbed. If this happens, there isn't enough stored for release next time. Enzyme levels can be too high and destroy many neurotransmitter molecules before they reach the receptor, or cut up so many that there is none available for re-uptake. Other kinds of molecules can block receptor sites, and defective neurons may not have the right number or type of receptors. In these cases, there may be enough neurotransmitter, but no parking spots for them.

Serotonin

Of the dozens of neurotransmitters already discovered, serotonin is currently still believed to be one of the best targets for influencing behavior problems. It is a neurotransmitter that is both important for directly controlling moods and behavior, and also for acting as a master chemical that regulates the activity of many other neurotransmitters. In contrast to other neurotransmitters, which are concentrated in a few specific areas of the brain, serotonin producing neurons are found in many key locations, such as the limbic system, the part of the brain that controls emotion and impulsivity. Serotonin has other effects throughout the body. It is found in blood platelets as well as in the digestive tract.

Among the many conditions that are associated with low serotonin levels are aggression, anxiety and depression. Manifestations of low serotonin may vary from dog to dog, due to individual biochemistry and histories. Serotonin levels can often be boosted with drugs and/or through the use of nutrition and/or supplements.

Meds

There are four basic types of drugs that have effects on the serotonin system. The oldest type is the tricyclics such as amitriptyline (Elavil). These work by reducing serotonin re-uptake (thus achieving a higher net level of serotonin in the synapse). They also affect the re-uptake of other important neurotransmitter systems and it is thought that these other actions are what produce side effects reported in humans such as dry mouth, nausea, increased heart rate, dizziness, constipation, and fatigue. It is unknown exactly to what extent these are present in dogs.

Another class of drugs is the monoamine oxidase (MAO) inhibitors. They work by slowing down the activity of the enzyme (monoamine oxidase) that breaks down monoamine neurotransmitter molecules (like serotonin) as they float around in the synapse. Just like tricyclics, MAO inhibitors also act on other neurotransmitters and have a high risk of side effects.

The third class of drugs is the serotonin re-uptake inhibitors (SRI's). They inhibit serotonin re-uptake, allowing more serotonin to be available to bind to receptor sites. Drugs from this class that affect only the serotonin system are known as selective serotonin re-uptake inhibitors (SSRI's). Examples are Prozac, Paxil, Zoloft and Luvox. Because SSRI's affect just the serotonin system, they are thought by many to be less likely to cause as severe side effects as tricyclics or MAO inhibitors.

There are a number of agents in new classes that have not yet been used much in dogs, such as Wellbutrin. There is one drug, BuSpar (buspirone hydrochloride), that has been used in dogs to treat anxiety. It is an anxiolytic agent that is not chemically or pharmacologically related to benzodiazepines (like Valium and Klonopin), anti-depressants, or barbiturates. It acts by boosting dopamine and noradrenaline while reducing serotonin. Selegiline (Anipryl) is a MAOI that has been successfully prescribed for canine cognitive disorder. Its action is to increase dopamine while regulating pituitary ACTH.

Natural Remedies—Supplying the Body with More Building Blocks

The body produces these brain chemicals from amino acids found in proteins in food. To produce serotonin, the body converts the amino acid tryptophan into 5-HTP, and then converts 5-HTP into serotonin. For decades in the US, tryptophan (specifically the commercially manufactured version, L-tryptophan) was used as a treatment for problems associated with depleted serotonin. In 1989, an outbreak of EMS—a serious immune response that killed nearly thirty people—was tracked to tainted L-tryptophan supplements and the FDA banned it. Although the EMS outbreak was traced to a single manufacturer whose production method resulted in contamination, rather than to the use of L-tryptophan per se, tryptophan remained off the market in the US, while still being available in Canada. The tryptophan recall has since been re-evaluated, and in the meantime, serotonin's more immediate precursor, 5-HTP, has become increasingly popular. Tryptophan rich foods include bananas, milk, grapefruit, and turkey.

Melatonin, a hormone produced by the pineal gland, has generated some interest among dog people for the occasional management of separation anxiety. It's important to note that the effects of long-term use of melatonin are not known and so is never advised. The herb St. John's Wort has been used for centuries in Europe to treat human depression. There is some European evidence that the key ingredient, hypericin, inhibits serotonin re-uptake in some people and that other compounds in St. John's Wort, such as flavonoids, might provide other therapeutic benefits. A problem associated with natural remedies is that their quality is unregulated and their efficacy unclear. Dog owners are in an even more uncertain situation as most of these remedies have next to no published research about their effects in dogs.

Desensitization to Veterinarian Visits

Dear Jean,

My dog, Katalin, is so dear to me I can barely find words. I rescued her at age five and she is now eleven. She is a Vizsla who has done some obedience and agility, but is now retired to long walks and cuddles on the sofa. The problem is that ever since I've had her, she has been terrified of going to the

KEY CONCEPTS
Desensitization
Counter-conditioning
Situational anxiety

vet. She trembles, pants, salivates, and tries to escape, even if it's just a check-up. Although she has never tried to bite the staff, I am worried she eventually might, as that is how out of her mind she is. The last time we went, the vet had given me a sedative to administer to her beforehand. It made her look drunk, but she seemed just as petrified, perhaps even more from being in this weird altered state while forced to the place she so dreads. I am at a complete loss as to how to help her, but desperately want to. As she gets older I want to be on top of whatever age-related health conditions she develops and dread putting her through this more frequently. Is there anything I can do for her?

First of all, I must commend you for wanting to alleviate your dog's anxiety. Legions of dogs are uncomfortable about vets and groomers, but must tough it out their entire lives. My heart breaks to see anxious old dogs put through things that scare them. There is a technique, desensitization and counter-conditioning, which has a good track record for ameliorating situational anxiety like Katalin experiences at the vet. It is extremely labor-intensive, so requires some considerable patience on your part, but the result should be well worth the effort.

The procedure involves exposing Katalin to a reduced intensity of experience at the veterinarian and pairing this less awful version with some fabulous thing, like a favorite game or extremely, super-duper high value heavy artillery treat (no plain old cookies please—use something like diced grilled chicken, freeze dried liver or pecorino Romano cheese, something she never, ever gets in other contexts—I repeat, it must be the good stuff). After repeating exposure at the reduced level and pairing with the super-treats, you then very, very gradually increase the intensity until you've worked your way up to her being comfortable with the real thing.

To accomplish this, it's important you choose a period of time where she won't have to actually go for a real visit. This would slow down your progress. Then, get permission from your veterinarian to drop by a couple of times a week, to hang out for half an hour or so. On the first visit, you have to find the level your dog can cope with without any trembling or panting. This will probably mean outside the door. Hang around outside and, every few minutes, make a short trip with her into the waiting room for a few seconds and then leave again to hang around outside. Give her a few treats in the waiting room or, if she won't take them there, right away once you get outside. Keep going in and out, proving to her that nothing more is going to happen. The goal is for her to learn that the trip to the waiting room means she's about to get a treat (and not a shot!). As she relaxes and starts to like the game, extend the amount of time in the waiting room. I recommend going from a few seconds to ten seconds. Do several trials at ten until she is clearly very interested in and anticipating the treat, as well as exhibiting no trepidation about being there. Once this is solid, try twenty seconds, then thirty, then a minute. From here go up in one minute increments. When you can be in the waiting room for five or ten minutes and she will happily take treats there, it's time to start visiting the treatment rooms (you'll need permission from your vet for this, however most vets are happy to have their dog clients worked on this way).

Repeat this same procedure, moving from the waiting room to the treatment room in short bursts. When she can hang out happily in the treatment room for ten minutes, it's time to introduce some staff. The staff at vet clinics are extremely busy, but should be happy to pop into the room you're in on their way by, give your girl a pat and a treat, and then get back to what they were doing.

All this may take a dozen visits, possibly more for your golden girl. In between visits, you're going to practice three things: restraining her like a veterinary technician, playing doctor with her like a veterinarian, and putting her up on tables to simulate the exam table. Only once these things have been practiced separately will you combine them, first at home and then at the clinic.

To best simulate one of those vet-tech restraining headlocks, firmly hold out one of her forelegs as though they're about to take blood. Do it briefly, like a game, and then give her one of those incredible treats. Once again, work your way gradually up to the real thing, always building on success. The most important rule is to not make things harder unless she is 100% comfortable and clearly loving the treats. If ever she becomes less interested in the treats or seems worried, back off to the last level at which she was comfortable and go more slowly.

When she's a star at both visits to the premises and being poked, prodded and restrained by you, it's time to combine them in a real visit. Always pack your super treats and dispense them liberally throughout. Ask for permission to accompany her into any treatment room, explaining why. If ever you have advance notice that she is to have some particular procedure done, prepare her for it by practicing whatever particular restraining hold or poke she will have to endure.

If this all sounds too daunting, another option for you is to find a veterinarian who does house calls. This could give you a fresh start—the first brief visit or two of the new doctor, for instance, would be just to meet your dog, give her some treats, show her the equipment, but not do any remotely invasive doctor stuff. Although not all procedures can be accomplished without going to a hospital, this will reduce the number of times she has to be so stressed.

Separation Anxiety

Dear Jean,

Our English Setter, Hugh, is a retired conformation champion. He is five years old and well mannered around the house when we are home. The problem is when we leave him alone for any length of time. He chews and digs at the front door frame, sometimes even breaking his nails and making his paws bleed. He is long past the puppy stage and gets thirty to sixty minutes of exercise per day. We got him nearly two years ago and he was fine until a month and a half ago, when we boarded him with neighbors for a week while we took a cruise. Within a week of getting back, he began the chewing and digging. He is in excellent health and has no other behavior problems. It seems clear to me he has separation anxiety, but a trainer friend says that diagnosis is currently out of vogue. What is the current thinking and what can we do for him?*

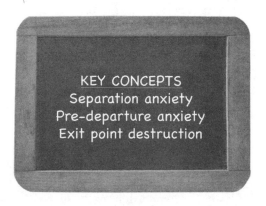

KEY CONCEPTS
Separation anxiety
Pre-departure anxiety
Exit point destruction

There still is and likely always will be a bona fide disorder called separation anxiety. I think your trainer friend might have a finger too strongly adhered to the pulse of popular media, which brought sep-anx into people's living rooms via a couple of high profile segments on prime time television shows some years ago. Shortly thereafter, everybody's dog who misbehaved when alone had separation anxiety. Inevitably, a backlash ensued: no, no, stop being so new-agey, they don't have separation anxiety, they're just being naughty.

Throughout these popular pendulum swings, behavior counselors in the trenches continued to diagnose and treat problems of both stripe. The truth is that owner-absent problems— specifically, some combination of destructiveness, vocalization, and house-soiling— can occur in dogs who are just being dogs and killing time while alone, or in dogs with separation anxiety, a severe disorder with a specific treatment approach.

The tricky bit is that the two problems can present similarly. For instance, the fact that the dog misbehaves solely when left alone can be a feature of both garden-variety misbehavior and sep-anx. As Ian Dunbar has pointed out, dogs without anxiety disorders quickly learn that their owners attack them when they chew or eliminate in the house. This can backfire if the dog becomes inhibited about eliminating or acting like a dog in the owner's presence at all. The result is a dog that desperately holds on to bladder and bowels while on walks and then, once the owner leaves, relieves himself. The owner may then interpret the problem as spite at being left alone and then punish the dog on their arrival home. This ultra-late punishment can have the ironic effect of contributing to a bona fide anxiety disorder, as it is crazy-making to be punished dozens if not hundreds of behaviors after the fact. The dog now has two reasons to eliminate when alone: it's the only time it's safe to do so and his panic attack makes him lose bladder and bowels. This same vicious cycle can play out for chewing.

What Is Separation Anxiety?

Part of our enchantment with dogs is their capacity to bond. The idea has been floated that separation anxiety is a form of hyper-bonding. In support of this is the observation that separation anxiety is often triggered by a temporary disruption in owner access. Experiences such as being boarded for extended periods, the death or departure of a key family member, and re-homing often kick it off. The theory is that when a susceptible dog has an important bond broken and then has a subsequent opportunity to re-bond, the new bond is tighter, desperately so. Not all dogs are susceptible—in fact, most never develop separation anxiety, sailing through potential trigger experiences. It's currently impossible to identify susceptible animals in advance. Another interesting fact about separation anxiety is that it is typically presented without other behavior problems. Sep-anx dogs are often model dogs when they're not left alone.

Differential Diagnosis

The easiest way to diagnose bona fide separation anxiety is to screen for features that are unique to it. Some common sep-anx features—behavior problems that manifest exclusively when the dog is alone, presence of vocalization, arrival elation, and shadowing the owner around the house—can also be present in dogs without the disorder. The cardinal symptoms that are more exclusive to sep-anx are:

- **Pre-departure anxiety**. Dogs learn tip-offs to important environmental events—leashes mean walks and the cookie cupboard means possible cookies. They also learn the sequence of events that lead up to being left alone, an extremely important event for a dog with separation anxiety. This is most apparent if there is a set ritual the owner engages in leading up to exiting the house. At some point during the morning routine, the dog may start to pant, pace, appear lethargic, salivate, tremble, hide, or refuse to eat. Owners may describe them as mopey, agitated, or sometimes even "resentful."

- **Exit-point destruction**. The destructiveness of dogs with separation anxiety has a different flavor than that of dogs engaged in recreation. They are trying to escape rather than pass time and so direct chewing and digging at doors and windows.

- **Self-injury**. The same desperation that prompts sep-anx dogs to go for exit points makes them sometimes do so to the point of hurting themselves. Broken teeth or bleeding paws or muzzle are extremely diagnostic of separation anxiety. Sep-anx dogs left in secure crates (not usually a good idea) sometimes salivate to the point of soaking themselves by the time the owner arrives home.

- **Anorexia**. Dogs with separation anxiety are too upset to eat or engage chew toys while alone. The anorexia can bleed backwards to the pre-departure ritual as well. If you're not sure whether Hugh has this symptom, leave in plain view, or in his bowl, some very attractive treat such as cheddar cheese cubes or roast chicken, and see if he consumes it during your absence. A typical sep-anx dog will not touch the goodies while alone, but vacuum them within a short time of the owner's arrival home, once the anxiety has abated. The dog clearly knew they were there.

Hugh's doorframe destruction and bleeding paws strongly suggest separation anxiety. You can firm up his diagnosis with an anorexia test and consideration of whether there is any pre-departure anxiety evident. Another way to firm up a tentative or unsure diagnosis is to videotape the dog for the first hour (often the worst time) while alone, to witness whether he's having a good time or a panic attack. The onset of Hugh's sep-anx being after a boarding stay is classic.

There is a behavior modification procedure with an excellent track record for separation anxiety. And, one good piece of fallout from the popularization of the diagnosis is the increased availability of medications to use along with the behavior modification. Next we'll look at treatment using this two-pronged approach.

The goal of treatment is for the dog to be able to be left alone without anxiety. There is no controversy regarding what does and doesn't work in this regard. Punishing dogs for misbehaviors stemming from the anxiety—whether after the fact punishments or somehow well timed—is ineffective and inhumane. Routine behavior problem management, such as use of confinement, and increased exercise and stimulation, usually can't dent severe separation anxiety once it's up and running. The treatment of choice is desensitization and counter-conditioning (D&C) to owner departures. It's been reported that D&C is more successful when supplemented with a program of structuring interactions with the dog so that he must perform a simple command before being fed, having a door opened for him, being patted or given attention, so it is worth adding to the regime.

Desensitization is a technique originally developed for people with phobias. It has since also proven useful for dogs with certain fear and aggression problems. In the case of separation anxiety, desensitization involves exposing the dog to a length of absence that he can handle without any anxiety and then gradually increasing that length up a carefully constructed hierarchy. The dog is successful every step of the way, so, in well-executed desensitization, at no point does the dog experience the original anxiety.

Counter-conditioning, an application of Pavlovian conditioning, is usually used in conjunction with desensitization. Dogs who have negative emotions about something (in this case, being left alone) can have a new emotional response conditioned to counter the existing distress. Successful D&C changes the dog's association with alone time from The Abyss to No Problem (desensitization) and Actually Kind of Good (counter-conditioning).

Dogs with separation anxiety usually succumb to panic attacks within a few minutes to half an hour of their owners' departures, so the length of absence on the first rung of the hierarchy must be under this. The procedure is quite simple: the owner rehearses many absences under the dog's anxiety threshold. If the dog continues to demonstrate no angst before departures and minimal interest in returns, the training is on safe ground and the next level can be commenced.

To condition a new, relaxed and happy association, a novel and enticing chew-toy, such as a stuffed Kong™, can be supplied prior to each departure and removed upon arrival. Along with its potency as a counter-conditioning stimulus, such a toy comes to signal: "don't worry—this absence will be of a length you can handle" to the dog (especially helpful for Plan B, below). It also provides a useful gauge of whether the dog has crossed the anxiety threshold. Not all owners are skilled at reading signs of low-grade anxiety, so it's useful to provide owners the clearer task of judging whether the dog is all over the Kong.

I've come across various rules of thumb for increments to build absence length tolerance and what follows is a composite of these:

- For the first two minutes, go up in 1—5 second increments, varied.

- From two to ten minutes, go up in fifteen to thirty second increments, throwing in a few one to five second absences.

- From ten to thirty minutes, go up in one minute increments, throwing in the odd five to fifteen second absences to mix it up.

- From thirty to ninety minutes, go up in ten to fifteen minute increments, throwing in some fifteen to thirty second absences (these short trials should not be omitted—they take literally seconds and plenty of them does no harm so they can be used as liberally as the client likes).

- From ninety minutes to a full day, go up in fifteen to thirty minute increments, still throwing in the short mini-absences on a regular basis.

- For maintenance, retain the throwing in of "easy question"—extremely brief—absences in day to day life, as well as keeping departures and arrivals low key emotionally, and the work-to-eat and work-for-attention regimen.

Many dogs with separation anxiety start descending into anxiety during the owner's getting-ready-to-leave routine. In these cases, the owner must commence desensitization to the cues that kick off the anxiety before attempting absences of even a second or two. These tip-off cues might be late in the sequence—owner picking up keys or reaching for door; or early—owner rising early, showering, and putting on work clothes (which predicts an absence), rather than sleeping in (which predicts the owner being home at least for a while). Once the dog is desensitized to pre-departure cues, the absences can begin, using the template above.

The ideal is for the dog to not experience absences over his anxiety threshold for the duration of treatment. This means never leaving the dog alone for longer than has been reached in treatment sessions to date. For many owners this is not at all realistic, and for these cases we go to Plan B.

Plan B

If the dog must sometimes be left alone for longer than he can tolerate, a clear distinction has to be made to—with luck—protect the progress in treatment sessions. The dog needs to be able to tell safe (treatment) length absences from anxiety-eliciting (unavoidable over-threshold length) absences in day to day life. If the same "picture" leads sometimes to the safe length absence and sometimes not, the former is poisoned by the latter and the anxiety disorder remains. To avoid this, don't lie to the dog—if it's going to be an anxiety-eliciting length of absence, signal it ahead of time. If it's going to be under threshold, signal this. The counter-conditioning Kong can help in this regard along with varying the routine to further help the dog discriminate.

For example, in a case I worked on a few years ago, the dog's owners put a plexiglas barrier over the front door prior to departures to minimize the damage to the moldings around the door as well as protect the dog. This became a cue to the dog that he was about to be left alone. These particular clients were unable to completely eliminate too-long absences for the duration of treatment. So, when they were exiting for an unavoidable, over-threshold length of time, they put up their Plexiglas as usual. When they were practicing their D&C exercises, they did not put up the Plexiglas, and provided a stuffed Kong. Over time, the safe, treatment "picture" predicted sessions with absences of a length that enabled the clients to live their normal life, so they simply threw out their Plexiglas. Life had become the safe session. The drawback to Plan B is that it doesn't work in all cases. Some dogs simply do better if they are protected from having any more panic attacks at all.

Medication

The odds of success in treatment of separation anxiety can be improved by using anti-anxiety medications in conjunction with the behavior modification outlined above. One drug, a tri-cyclic antidepressant, clomipramine hydrochloride (Clomicalm), has passed FDA standards for safety and efficacy for the treatment of separation anxiety in dogs. Other agents, such as amitriptyline (Elavil, also a tri-cyclic) and fluoxetine (Prozac, in the SSRI class) are also used, but their usage is considered off-label, which can dissuade veterinarians from prescribing them. All these medicines take up to six weeks to confer benefit, so a decision must be made between the behavior practitioner, veterinarian, and client, whether to start the D&C immediately while waiting for the meds to kick in, or get the meds on board and up to blood level before starting the behavior mod. Some veterinarians opt to use sedatives, on a short-term basis at the beginning of treatment, to buy time for the anti-anxiety drug to kick in. There have been some tantalizing reports of melatonin, a pineal gland secretion given in supplement form, for short-term management of over-threshold absences, however safety (especially long-term) and efficacy research is yet to surface for this.

Do Dogs Pick Up Their Owners' Prejudices?

Dear Jean,

A supplier at work was telling me about his dog who has this quirk. The dog growls at and avoids being patted by people of Asian descent. As he kept talking, I got the impression that this person was himself maybe a bit of a bigot and so I got to wondering whether the dog is acting out his owner's prejudices. I always thought one of the great things about dogs was that they don't discriminate the way people do. Do they?

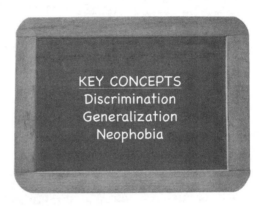

KEY CONCEPTS
Discrimination
Generalization
Neophobia

Dogs do discriminate, but not in all the ways that we do.

The word discriminate, when used in everyday conversation, usually means considering a person or category of people to be less worthy and then proceeding to treat them badly. In western society, discrimination on the basis of race, sex, age, ethnicity, body size, or mobility is considered universally repugnant and our laws and morals reflect this. History does seem to have demonstrated that humans are prone to be prejudiced, however, though whether it's through our biology or culture (i.e., indoctrination and modeling) or both is a hot and far from laid to rest topic.

The word discriminate also has a very precise, techie meaning in the psychology of animal learning. An animal that can discriminate can tell the difference between two or more things and then employ that ability to respond differently. A dog who has learned that "sit" means "put rear on floor" and "down" means "put rear and elbows on floor" is performing an auditory discrimination. If the cues were hand signals, it would be a visual discrimination. A rodent pest that has learned to avoid the smell of poisonous bait discovered on a dead colleague is performing an olfactory discrimination task.

Depending on its particular ecology, a given species of animal will have more or less ability to discriminate using its various senses. For example, many species of foraging birds have terrific visual acuity—they can tell the difference between tiny pebbles and tiny edible things. Dogs famously have amazing olfactory discrimination ability, which is why they can be used to detect drugs, bombs, mines, cancer, etc.

The extrapolation of responding to stuff that is not identical, but in some way similar, to an original stimulus is known as generalization. Let's say in an auditory discrimination task, a dog learns to associate a tone at 400 Hertz with food, and so salivates when he hears the tone. The dog doesn't salivate to the 1812 Overture or to just any old sound. But a single tone at 450 hertz elicits some salivation response, typically less than the response to 400 Hertz. Ditto the response to 350 Hertz tones. And then less still—but still somewhat—to 500 and 300 Hertz. As the frequency departs from the original trained stimulus, the degree of responding drops off in a lovely bell curve known as a generalization gradient.

We humans are master generalizers. For instance, we will place solidly in the category "men with beards" men with goatees, blond beards, wizard-y gray beards, a photo of a man with a beard, and Santa Claus. In fact we're more likely to place Santa in the category with a goateed man than a woman with an identical goatee to the man, even if her height, weight and hair style were identical to a given man with a beard. Language gives us the ability to employ specific parameters as the relevant to the criteria defining a category, and these parameters can be astoundingly abstract (ponder for a minute the category "geeks"). Dogs don't have nearly this degree of flexibility with regard to how a category is defined. They do pretty well on demographics, however, which brings us back to your question.

It's not been researched, but it's the overwhelming experience of dog owners that dogs readily employ sex, race, and age to categorize people. But although dogs discriminate—tell the difference between—categories of people, their category specific reactions are not governed by value judgments the way ours often are. The kind of cognition necessary to categorize people based on abstract concepts like moral superiority, being in the "right" religious or ethnic group, or aligned with one's own values are likely unique to humans. Dogs categorize on two bases:

1. Novelty of a person or category of people.
2. Good or bad experiences with a person or category of people.

Some dogs, through selective breeding, are extremely sociable toward new people regardless of category. Other dogs, also through selective breeding (sometimes deliberately and sometimes by a failure of omission), are socially neophobic to some degree—inclined to not be sociable with new people, the degree sometimes being influenced by how far a new person departs from the demographics of the dog's owner or very familiar people (the peak of the dog's generalization gradient). If a dog has never encountered men with beards (notably as a puppy), for instance, and is a susceptible (prone to social neophobia) individual, the dog may react fearfully or aggressively to men with beards. Ditto if the dog has had bad experiences with men with beards. Double ditto if the first time (i.e., novelty) a socially shy dog encounters a man with a beard she has a bad experience. People are like dogs in this regard; phobias can develop based on bad experiences and then generalize to entire categories.

So the bottom line is: dogs absolutely discriminate in the "can tell the difference" way, but any untoward responding they do is not due to "considering this group less worthy" or other high concept. This means your colleague's dog isn't employing any value judgment about Asian people. He's growling either because he didn't encounter enough of them (especially as a puppy) and so is not socialized to them and/or had a bad experience.

A very likely mechanism for what might appear to us to be a dog "picking up" her owner's prejudice is that owners who don't like certain categories of people may avoid them, thus resulting in poor or non-existent socialization to that category. Another possible, though less likely mechanism, is Pavlovian conditioning. If the owner getting stressed in the past makes the owner smell a certain way and that smell has led to bad things for the dog, the dog would learn that that smell predicts bad news. If the presence of certain types of people then caused the owner to be stressed and smell that way, it's possible the dog might then acquire a negative emotional response to that category of people.

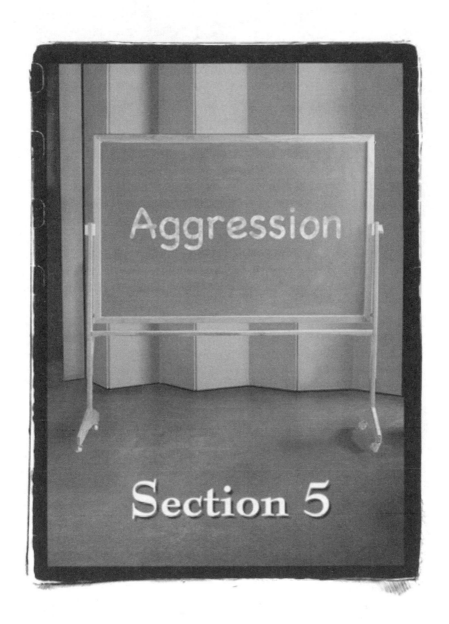

Aggression

Section 5

The Dog Bite Epidemic

Dear Jean,

I am not a dog person, although I have owned dogs. I read in the paper last year about an elderly woman near Los Angeles having both arms amputated by her great grandson's Pit Bull. Shortly before this, I read of a Doberman that killed someone in New York State. My neighbor's dog growled and barked at my husband when he poked his head over the fence this weekend. These incidents seem to be on the rise. With all due respect, what are you dog people doing about it?

KEY CONCEPTS
Folk statistics
Hazards of everyday life
Dread factor

This is an explosive topic, but an interesting one. The interest lies in how different the reality is from the public perception of how dangerous dogs are to people and whether this is worsening. Meaningful discussion about dogs and public health is retarded by: 1) the lumping of routine dog threat behavior and non-damaging bites together with the extraordinarily rare events of fatalities and serious maulings (this is like lumping human arguments and office politics together with aggravated assault and murder); and 2) the stupendously exaggerated estimation of one's own risk of serious dog attack based on the prevalence of stories about them in the media.

Dogs are, compared to other "hazards" we accept without question in our society, fantastically safe. My friend and colleague, Janis

Bradley, thoroughly researched this topic for her amazing book, *Dogs Bite But Balloons and Slippers Are More Dangerous*. In it she compares dogs to everything from kitchen utensils and water buckets to strollers, Christmas trees, balloons, and marbles. To these items they compare favorably. They compare even more favorably to things like swimming pools, bicycles, and playground equipment. And, when it comes to the heavy-duty statistic-makers in our society, she writes, "dogs can never compete as hazards with fathers or mothers or sisters or brothers or aunts or uncles or friends…"

Bradley underscores her point about how vanishingly rare fatal dog attacks are by comparing them to the "universal cliché" of being struck by lighting. We are each "five times as likely to be killed by a bolt of lightning—not just struck by one, mind you—killed" than to be killed by a dog or dogs. Considering that less than 20% of lightning strikes are fatal, this makes being struck by lightning twenty-five times more likely than being the victim of a fatal dog mauling. If the risk by exposure is then considered—there is one dog for every four or five people in the United States for instance, and most of these dogs encounter several people every day of their lives—dogs are almost incalculably safe.

And, contrary to shrieking newspaper headlines, dog-related deaths are not trending upwards. The rate has remained astonishingly steady over all the decades that records have been kept. Bradley surmises that this may indicate that the floor has been reached, i.e., that the rate is as low as it could conceivably get. In fact, she cautions that well-meant swells to "do more" after every headline-grabbing incident might not only do nothing (save robbing resources from elsewhere), but rock a boat that is currently at rock bottom: "Basic systems theory teaches us that it is perilous to change the system to eradicate the exception, and dog bite deaths are about as exceptional as it gets. It is perilous because when you change large scale situations to prevent extremely rare events, you cannot even begin to predict what other aberrant, or even widespread, events may pop up."

When it comes to bites at the kitchen-injury level, however, dog bites are relatively frequent. What do I mean by "kitchen-injury" level? Injuries are classified on a scale from one to six, with Level

One defined as quick recovery with no lasting impairment and six defined as likely fatal. Ninety-nine percent of all treated dog bites fall into the "one" category. For comparison purposes, Bradley discusses falls, the most common type of injury, which average a four rating, defined as requiring weeks or months for full healing or some lasting minor impairment.

So what about frequency? Based on inferences from the available research, for instance, it is often quoted that half of all children will be bitten by dogs at some point and that every human who lives to the age of sixty will be bitten at least once. This qualifies low-level dog bites as mundane events. Absurdly mundane, according to Bradley, who points out that a huge proportion of adults will also nick themselves with paring knives countless times during their lives, and that "something close to 100% of kids fall off their bikes multiple times without injury." What's amazing about dog bites is that we are grimly trying to count them: "There is no other such phenomenon that anyone even attempts to study when it doesn't produce physical harm." In other words, no one talks about the paper-cut epidemic, the chef's knife injury epidemic, or the falling in bathtub epidemic. Why do dogs get to have "an epidemic" when five gallon buckets, which are more dangerous, don't?

Barry Glassner, a sociology professor at USC and author of *The Culture of Fear*, points to the disproportional media coverage given to certain kinds of events relative to the "near invisibility" of other kinds of injury that seriously hurt and kill people. Dogs meet criteria for what Glassner calls "cultural scapegoating." Bradley puts it well when she notes that dogs (or perhaps their "irresponsible owners") might qualify as "unambiguous villains that allow us to distance ourselves from responsibility for the real problems in our society."

Another reason for humans' exaggerated fear of dog bites is our evolutionary heritage. Just as we inherited a craving for fat and sugar that served us well in our distant past amidst dietary scarcity and now is maladaptive, we inherited a preparedness for fearing certain environmental elements, such as animals with big teeth. These were genuine and prevalent concerns back then. Now they are not, but we can't seem to shake the feeling, nor replace it with one that would be more adaptive, such as, say, motor vehicles at high speed. Dogs have higher "dread factor" than cars.

Rational discussions about routine dog bites, and especially about serious dog attacks, can get derailed when they raise the hackles of dog bite victims and their advocates who feel their suffering is being minimized. I dread seeing Janis misunderstood and attacked on Larry King Live or in print, which I fear is her destiny. But I hope that cooler heads will ultimately prevail.

Aggression Prognosis Estimates

Dear Jean,

Buster, our rescued Old English Sheepdog, is affection-ate and handsome, but also extremely complex. When we first got him, it took us months to win his trust enough so that he'd let us brush him and trim his nails. The rescue organiza-tion said he was likely abused. He's a bit growly and snappy

KEY CONCEPTS
Test-retest reliability
Inter-tester reliability
Predictive validity
Reporting errors
Prognosis assessment
Bite inhibition

when we reprimand him or take things away and, if pushed, bites us. He has in fact bitten us an embarrassing number of times (our feelings were hurt more than our hands luckily!) in dramatic confrontations over dirty socks. Last week he chewed my husband's best shoes to bits. We decided to get our heads out of the sand and get some professional help.

We ended up taking him to three different dog behavior experts to have him assessed. One said he was a status-seeking dog, would always be this way, but that we could keep him in check with obedience and certain lifestyle changes. Another play-fought with him, which he loves, and then remarked that he "lacked boundaries" with him during the assessment. Because of this, he said, Buster was almost certainly going to seriously bite someone sooner or later so should be put to sleep immedi-ately. We were agog. The third flipped him on his back and held him down. Buster wouldn't go near her afterwards and we felt very upset and left the office.

*We are frankly extremely confused by these opinions and assessment
procedures. Is he an abuse survivor? A social climber? Non-respectful of
boundaries? What confidence should we have in these opinions? Can his
behavior be changed or is it his basic personality that is the problem?*

Dog behavior is an area with an astounding scarcity of scientific
research addressing basic questions such as how to predict future
behavior, aggressive and otherwise. This knowledge void has created
fertile ground for all manner of explanatory constructs and tests of
presumed immutable character traits. And, as you've found, professional behavior counselors may have wildly diverse opinions and
self-invented classification systems, yet pass these off as gospel to
their clients. Imagine if dentists did it this way!

There are, at present, no dog assessment procedures that are strong
on the two critical test evaluation yardsticks of reliability and validity. Test-retest reliability is the achieving of a replicable result in
multiple administrations of the test over time. If I test a dog today
and again in a month, are the results the same? Inter-tester reliability refers to the achieving of similar results on the test with different
testers. If three people conduct the same test on the dog, do they all
get the same results? Validity is the test's ability to predict behavior
in the real world. Given the notoriously weak track records of tests
in these areas, it's safe to say these consultants, and others who read
a lot into behavior evaluations and temperament tests, are on shaky
ground and ought to have been more circumspect. They may even
be using procedures that have not undergone reliability or validity
testing at all!

You raise a behavior vs. personality question that has interesting
nature-nurture shades and I will defer that discussion in Section 6
on Genetics and Evolution that follows. The other, more practical question is that of prognosis assessment, i.e., how can one tell
whether a dog with an aggression problem is a good candidate
for behavior modification? With reliability and validity problems
plaguing currently available behavior tests, the other remaining
avenue for prognosis information is history-taking.

History is usually obtained by client interview. The value of history
is that it gets at both context and trend. There's a saying that goes:

behavior predicts behavior. What a dog does today in a certain context is the best predictor of what he will do in that same context tomorrow. This is thought to be part of the reliability and validity obstacles in behavior evaluations. Does a tester represent all people to a dog? Do the test items adequately simulate real-life contexts? In the case of history, these bases are better covered and, if trend is added to that, predictions became firmer. What a dog did the last three weeks, three months, or three years in a certain context is the best predictor of what he will do in that same context tomorrow.

The downside of history taking is reporting error. We have all heard the stories of enacted events in law school auditoriums and the wildly conflicting eye-witness accounts that ensue from the observing students, all given with great self-assurance. In the case of the reporting of dog bite incidents, this notoriously poor recall of critical event details is potentially compounded by the strong emotions involved and any vested interest an interview subject might have in subconsciously (or consciously) either inflating or deflating severity. These factors must always be kept in mind when taking history.

Prognosis assessments should incorporate thorough histories and, if necessary to complement or confirm, direct observations in the real contexts in which the problem occurs. This requires greater legwork than a typical temperament test, but avoids those lethal testing problems. In the case of acquired bite inhibition, a vital prognostic indicator, history is the only means one can utilize, as deliberately orchestrating a bite is ethically too difficult to justify.

Here are some key factors that are relevant to prognosis:

- **Degree of acquired bite inhibition (ABI)**. This is the degree of jaw pressure exerted when the dog inflicts a bite. ABI warrants thorough exploration, which I'll get to in a bit. In Buster's case, this would be considered good. He has bitten "an embarrassing number" of times without inflicting serious injury.

- **Client compliance issues**. There are enormous differences among clients with regard to their level of commitment, competence at assigned exercises, and ability to manage the dog between treatment sessions. Practitioners have observed over and over otherwise simple cases that do poorly with less compliant clients and more severe and complex cases that re-solve in the charge of stellar human clients. In your case, the fact that you sought three opinions and critically evaluated these would suggest you are neither taking this lightly nor expecting an easy, quick fix. A practitioner's careful interview-ing would elucidate your understanding of and willingness to comply with a modification regime. So, jury partially out on this.

- **Bite threshold.** This is the number and intensity of stimuli required to get the dog to bite. Does a dog that is uncomfort-able with strangers, for instance, bite if a stranger is passing at an oblique angle three feet away or must the stranger be a foot away facing the dog and reaching out a hand? In a food-bowl guarding case, does the dog charge and bite a family member who enters the kitchen, only when touched while eating, or when the bowl is grasped and removed? That em-barrassing number of bites flags Buster as quite possibly hav-ing a low bite threshold, depending on how cozy and heated the exchanges were prior to his biting over all those socks.

- **Presence of protracted warning signs.** Does the dog tense up, growl, snarl or air-snap (as Buster has done) when his buttons are being pushed or do still waters run deep? As with the other indicators already listed, avoiding serious offense during the course of treatment is germane. Every time the dog bites, especially if there is damage, the client is demoral-ized, the dog's rap sheet grows along with the potential liabil-ity of both practitioner, and client and treatment protocols are often compromised. A dog with good ABI, an on-the-ball client, high bite threshold, and a dog that advertises before biting are all potential lines of defense in this regard. The more that are present, the greater the chance of preventing mishap both during and between treatment sessions.

As appealing as it is to humans to apply adjectives and labels to dogs, a focus on observable, quantifiable behavior—what the dog is doing—yields both modification strategies and objective means to assess whether modification strategies are working. Let's look at bite inhibition in more detail.

Bite Inhibition

Acquired bite inhibition is likely the most significant prognostic
indicator in aggression. What makes ABI so crucial a factor are
ethics and liability considerations. Should a dog being worked on
re-offend during or between treatment sessions, or post-treatment,
ABI dictates the degree of damage done to whoever is bitten. Given
that 100% is hard to achieve when it comes to behavior, there is
thus a large ethical responsibility to protect the owner and the public. The potential liability to both owner and practitioner escalates
astronomically when dogs do significant damage when they bite,
especially when this is known ahead of time.

With all the strides forward that have been made in the behavior modification of aggression, altering ABI has proven virtually
impossible in an adult dog (there is some promising suggestion of
influence on ABI by the use of certain psychotropic medications,
however this is not yet well established). And, no studies exist on its
acquisition, i.e., why one dog bites softly and another with mutilat-
ing force under similar circumstances. The generally accepted view
in the dog behavior field is that ABI is a result of a genetic predisposition combined with certain early environmental influences. The
key early influence is thought to be interactions between puppies
in a litter as well as subsequent play-biting up to the age when
the dog's permanent teeth are fully erupted, between four and five
months of age.

If you observe a litter of puppies, their primary activity—when
not eating, sleeping, or eliminating—is biting other puppies. Their
sharp teeth inflict pain if a bite is too hard, in spite of the pup's
weak jaw muscles. Play is derailed—a rotten consequence for the
hard biter—and, over time, puppies learn to not bear down with
full force when biting. They rehearse this restraint over and over.
Adult dogs are then equipped to solve conflicts ritualistically rather
than bearing the expense of flat-out aggression in every encounter.
ABI is thus the cornerstone of aggression ritualization. Bite inhibition acquisition is also believed to be part of the function of the
ceaseless play fighting that takes place in the young of other social
predatory species, such as hyenas.

The current thinking is that if a puppy does not get adequate re-hearsal at biting softly, he is at risk of growing to adulthood with-out the capacity to inhibit his jaw force when biting under duress. This means that ABI can be installed in puppies, but not in adult dogs, which elevates its priority level in puppy education curricula. The study that cries out to be done is one where this hypothesis is tested out. A design whereby puppies were divided into groups, one receiving standard measures to address ABI and the other not, may be deemed unethical if the study's result is thought to be somewhat pre-ordained, as the control group would be deliberately set up to become hard-mouthed adults. A safer study design would be retrospective: to take careful histories of dogs with known adult ABI levels and correlate these with the kinds of interventions they received as puppies.

The other oft-discussed factor is breed. Akitas, Chows and, to a lesser extent, Springer Spaniels, for instance, are believed by some trainers to be harder biters (and in the case of Akitas and Chows, low on protracted warning). Again, no objective data to back this up. An interesting question is whether some individuals in the thought-to-be higher risk breeds are destined to have hard mouths regardless of efforts exerted in puppy-hood or whether additional attention will produce good ABI. My suspicion (and hope) is the latter. One of my primary projects with my Chow, Buffy, was to work diligently on her ABI as a puppy, and then to continue rehearsing her soft mouth with regular dog-dog play sessions and regular dog-human play-wrestling sessions that incorporate time out penalties for all bites that are not gentle. My hope is that should she ever bite, it will be with restraint.

When presented with an adult dog, assessing ABI involves taking a comprehensive history of all bites and noting who was bitten, on what part of their body, through what kind of clothing and what degree of damage was inflicted. Consider the difference in jaw pressure between an eighty-pound dog biting the face of a five year-old child and leaving a minor laceration and a lot of saliva and an eighty pound dog biting the calf of a forty year old man through denim jeans and leaving contusions that spread many inches beyond the margins of the bite. Phrases like a bite "breaking skin" or "drawing blood" give inadequate information. In the first case above, the dog "broke skin" and has good ABI, whereas the second dog did not and has poor ABI. Pressure exerted is the key factor, not "blood."

A complete bite history will usually yield a pressure trend. In many cases, however, there are no or not many bites on record so ABI is unknown. Some hints at ABI may be gleaned from a dogfight history and play-biting history, though these are vastly inferior to the information obtained from jaw pressure under duress with a person. Remember: behavior predicts behavior. A dog with a long, colorful history of clean (non-injurious) dogfights and regular bouts since puppy-hood of playfully mouthing people (when invited of course—this is obnoxious behavior to most people), is a rosier ABI prospect than one who injures other dogs during scraps and has never mouthed a person softly. It would be extremely valuable for behavior practitioners to know whether ABI is specific to people vs. to dogs or whether one can extrapolate bite severity information between these two targets. But, alas, this represents yet another area of logical speculation rather than scientific fact.

The final two areas of exploration in ABI assessment are the dog's early history and hints about jaw restraint in the way the dog accepts treats and cookies. Early history centers around whether the dog in question engaged in regular enough play-biting of other puppies, such as in his litter and at a puppy kindergarten class. Less favorable is a dog that was sequestered until after his permanent teeth were all in or, worst of all, was a singleton in his litter and thereafter did not play-bite any puppies.

Dogs vary greatly in how gently they take tidbits from human hands. Dogs who are very rough can have this modified with standard consequence-type training. The treat is withheld after the barracuda grab is marked with "ouch!" and the dog invited to keep trying again until he takes it more gently. With repetition, the dog eventually gets it right most of the time. This training, however, has no bearing on the dog's jaw pressure when he bites under duress, the so-far unmodifiable ABI. The question then is whether any ABI information can be gleaned from the dog's initial tendencies when taking treats. I don't know very many knowledgeable practitioners who would bet much either way here.

Resource Guarding in Puppies

Dear Jean,

I just got a new nine week-old Rottie puppy. He's stunning, smart, and generally friendly, but growls and snaps if I go near him while he's eating. He also does this to my adult Rotties. I've never seen this in a puppy so young. Is he some sort of lemon? Is he a dominant dog? Is there anything I can do? Help!

KEY CONCEPTS
Genetic component to aggression
Susceptibility to behavior modification
Desensitization hierarchy design
Conditioned emotional response

It is indeed alarming for most people to see frank aggression in puppies. In the case of resource guarding—food, bone, bed possessiveness—there is good news and bad news. The good news is you can start addressing it in a young, hopefully plastic, spongy puppy with weak jaws. The bad news is that there is some sentiment out there among trainers that aggression in puppies is an insidious sign of the problem having Deep Genetic Roots and therefore fruitless to tackle. I'm going to explore the whole nature-nurture debate a little later, but for now will simply say that there doesn't seem to be any overwhelmingly tidy correlation between behavior problems that are thought to have a strong genetic component and their susceptibility (or lack thereof) to behavior modification.

I recently had a similar case with my own foster puppy. Buffy, then a stray six week-old Chow, presented with object and food guarding against people and dogs. I elected not to touch the dog-dog issues, which is a relatively common approach. Her socialization and play skills were coming along nicely and she was developing good acquired bite inhibition. The guarding against people, however, needed to be actively resolved. The following is a summary of Buffy's food guarding exercise regime. Incidentally, Buffy also presented with socialization deficits and severe body handling problems, which were also addressed, as was her object guarding. The key to good hierarchy design is small enough incremental steps that at no point do you see the original guarding problem. In the case of a puppy such as this, there may actually be more aggressive increment jumps. I did a few other things in the can't-hurt-might-help category. These included impulse control (stay, off, and wait) and extra soft-mouth training.

Baseline
When approached while eating from her dish, Buffy would freeze and, if the approach continued, growl briefly and then lunge and snap. If touched while eating, she would growl simultaneous to whirling and biting. Due to the independent body-handling problem, this had to be partly resolved prior to combining it with food bowl exercises. Buffy did not guard an empty dish.

Hierarchy
Step 1 (day 1): Installment Feeding of Canned Food
I sat on the floor next to Buffy's dish and spooned in one mouthful. Once she had swallowed, I spooned the next mouthful into her dish. By the end of the second meal, she demonstrated a clear happy anticipatory orientation to my spoon hand after each swallow.

Step 2 (day 1-2): Overlap
This was essentially the same as Step 1 except that I added the next spoonful to her dish while she was still consuming, always a much dicier proposition. We did this for three meals without evidence of guarding seen.

Step 3 (day 2-3): Approach Overlap

I was now standing. I spooned larger amounts, withdrew two paces, re-approached, and added the next spoonful while Buffy was still consuming. This combined an approach with the overlap exercise. We stuck with this for three meals, at end of which time a Conditioned Emotional Response (CER) had become evident—Buffy wagged and looked up on approach. We then repeated the exercise for one more day (five small meals) with larger withdrawal distances and intervals.

Step 4 (day 4): Trumping

Now I spooned her entire puppy-sized ration into her bowl. I withdrew five paces, paused fifteen seconds, approached and added a (hidden) marble-sized dollop of goat cheese. I had pre-auditioned the goat cheese out of context and ascertained it to be in Buffy's Top Five All Time Foods. I withdrew to six paces and waited for Buffy to continue to consume—this was not immediate (typical of trumping—dog orients to handler rather than back to dish)—then repeated. On the third trial I got a clear CER—withdrawal from bowl on approach, orientation to me, and tail wag. Clever little thing.

Step 5 (day 4-6): Covering High Value Base

To up the ante, I tried some approaches while she was consuming a top food (bowl of treats), rather than normal meal ration level food. I trumped it with higher value stuff (gorgonzola). In two trials, I once again saw her happy anticipatory CER, a very rapid curve indeed.

Step 6 (day 4 onward): Cold Trials

To better simulate real life, I initiated random trumping. At least once per meal, from a random direction, at a random time, and with one of Buffy's top foods, I approached and added the bonus. Better than 80% of the time, I got an evident "yippee" CER. At no point did she guard.

Step 7 (day 8 onward): Generalization

I recruited my husband, colleagues in my office, and a neighbor to do some random trumps, with careful monitoring for any evidence of regression, including the absence of "yippee" CERs to their approach. Had this been an adult dog, the hierarchy—and, notably, a much more gradual one too—would have been recommenced at the beginning by each new recruit, with likely accelerated progress rate for each successive person.

Step 8 (day 15 onward): Body Handling

It was only here that I commenced patting, grabbing, or pushing her around while she was eating. In most cases this would come earlier (be incorporated into the resource-guarding trials), however with Buffy it took me this long to get the independent body-handling problem up to speed. The handling during eating exercise consisted of the body touch (later handling) followed by a trumping addition, repeated until the body touch/handling elicited the "yippee" CER. Buffy's CER consisted of a wag as well as orientation to my hand. If I stored the bonus in my other hand behind my back or my pocket and reached with a blank hand, she would wag and orient to my face.

Buffy is now on maintenance with a cold trumping or body handling trial usually once per meal and use of other people whenever an opportunity presents itself. I ended up adopting her.

You can throw in bowl removals if you like, rather than sticking with approaches and body handling. The principles are the same. Good luck with your Rottie!

Buffy Age 2 Update

Buffy has improved with strangers, and has never snapped at or bitten anyone, however this remains the one incompletely resolved issue. While she is comfortable in their proximity, Buffy will duck away and sometimes bark if a stranger suddenly reaches for her head. It takes her twenty to thirty seconds of warm-up to allow new people to pat her. I will continue to chip away at this, and fully realize that at age two, there may still be developmental changes in store that could erode all gains.

As an interesting aside on her resource guarding, I slacked off on maintenance exercises for several months in the hope that some guarding against people might re-appear, so that she could be used as a known-good-mouth guarding case for Academy students.

Interestingly, she wouldn't guard even in a very stacked scenario. I'll carry on with this experiment as well as her other original problems and report back in a year.

Buffy Age 3 Update

Although I feared that onset of social maturity might roll back some of the gains she had made in her comfort around strangers, resource guarding, body handling and relations with other dogs, I am relieved to report that she is holding steady and has even made modest gains.

Buffy is still not Golden Retriever-like in her affinity to new people, but she warms up faster and faster—now typically fifteen seconds (from thirty or more previously)—and has tolerated with aplomb various semi-invasive stranger handling situations this year. For instance, I brought her to a new vet to have her eyes checked for entropion (an eyelid disorder) and she was stellar during the exam, including headlock restraint. The veterinarian remarked on Buffy's nice exam manners.

A parade of repairmen came and went from my house this year as both air-conditioning and heating were chronically on the fritz. After doorbell barking, she greeted all Men In Uniforms Carrying Implements very nicely. She has also attended numerous parties and events—brimming with crowds of both people and dogs—and exhibited no aggression and loved every minute. She is indeed a party animal.

I am still experimenting with withholding maintenance exercises on her former food and object guarding, but so far haven't been able to nurse back any guarding. There was a glimmer of something at one party when a trainer friend stacked up a great scenario with high-value bone, but it fizzled thereafter. So she is still not usable as an Academy project.

Her dog-dog is the same: she has many regular playmates, dozens of acquaintances, and meets on average a few new dogs per week, in a forward, chow-y manner, but also well within normal range of dog social behavior. She demonstrated admirable tolerance of my neighbors' puppies—a Siberian and a Pit Bull—playing with both after setting limits with growls and restrained snaps. I have fostered and dog-sat various dogs without incident. She guards food from other dogs but this is, for me, just dog behavior.

I've started remedial work on her feet, the one body-handling/grooming area I neglected up until now (to date I have pretty much coerced her for nails and scissoring, which is extremely naughty of me). It's a fun shaping project, luckily, which keeps me on task. After eight five to ten minute sessions, she's to the point where she'll lie on her side and present her feet for scissoring (two or three snips per treat currently), and target the nail-trimmers with her nose.

My husband and I still play-wrestle with her several times per week. Her lifetime bite tally is still zero. I'll continue the foot handling exercises, the neglect of food and object guarding and report back next year, when she turns four.

Buffy Age 4 Update

Buffy has had mostly a stellar year. No resource guarding with people, no body handling problems, and she's even better with strangers than she was last year, though a sudden approach and hand-reach of a new person still causes a head-duck about half the time. Her dog-dog interaction is the same as it was at age three: she is more selective about playmates than she was when she was younger and has the occasional posturing incident or resource-related scrap with another dog. No dogs were hurt during these spats with the exception of a foster Pomeranian I had who sustained one puncture to his withers. The dog had a pre-existing skin condition and so ended up with an infection at the puncture site, which was an ordeal. Since then I am more cautious with her around small dogs. I did not work on her resource guarding, however she is remaining a non-guarder so still can't be a "case" for an Academy student to work on. I also admit to not working on her as diligently as I might in the other areas this year, with the exception of occasionally using her as a demo dog for various training exercises. I'll report back in a year.

Buffy Age 5 Update

Continued gains with strangers this year, including a major test when my (new to Buffy) in-laws were houseguests for two weeks with their children aged six months and three years. I supervised extremely closely the first few days and pretty diligently thereafter, had the three-year old give Buffy cheese and showed her how to get Buffy to sit. There were no incidents, including when the baby pulled a wad of hair out of her tail with one of those infant death grips(!). I use her as a stimulus dog for dog-dog cases as she is quite bullet-proof. I continue to omit food and object guarding maintenance exercises in the hopes of using her for an Academy student project, but to no avail. It might be the rehab was done too early or pure luck. My one concern now is her bilateral luxating patellas. She is anesthesia intolerant so I am managing her without surgery.

Buffy Age 6 Update

Buffy has had a pretty much perfect year. She is now immediately social with most new people she meets. Her body handling—with the exception of nail-clipping (doesn't threaten or bite me, but is Non-Compliant)—is really good. Loves brushing and combing, being scissored, having her teeth brushed, ears cleaned, being pilled, vet exams, pretty much anything. Jumps on the grooming table on a Good Knees day. It's a reminder to me that a little effort can go a long way if you have the luxury of working on a young puppy. She is mostly good with the scores of dogs she encounters every week, mostly doing cordial investigations, very occasionally playing. She has an evil streak which manifests as occasional over-rough play and occasional ambushing of dogs using toys or bones as bait or just for the sheer naughtiness of it. A couple of minutes of time out and she rethinks this sport usually for a good couple of months before again "buffing" some dog.

Resource Guarding Prevention

Dear Jean,

I teach puppy classes and my focus is on socialization to people, handling and gentling, manners and beginner obedience, carefully monitored playgroups, and confidence-building activities like puppy agility. In the homework there is mention of hanging out with the dog while he eats, but 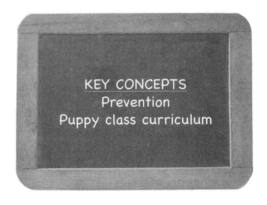 *I don't know how many, if any, of the students comply with this. So, I'd like to add some food-bowl work or other aggression prevention activities to the class itself. Any ideas?*

Puppy class curriculum choices are the toughest—there are so many worthy things to cram into the time allotted. You've hit the major bases beautifully and I love the idea of including some anti-aggression exercises, as odds are that some puppies in every class might start guarding at some point. It's a fair assumption that early intervention will either stave it off or help create smoother sailing in a treatment regime later on. Plus, if the owners have seen it done in a demo and practiced it themselves in class, you are likely to get better retention of the specifics than if it's assigned only as a homework extra.

Here are a few suggestions for class-friendly resource-guarding prevention activities.

1. Chew-toy sharing and exchanges during down-time. Sit on the floor with a puppy you have pre-auditioned to be interested in a chew toy such as a pig's ear, rawhide, bully-stick, or Greenie™. Hold the toy at angles advantageous to the dog (most dogs seem to appreciate this). Point out that many dogs have some natural instincts to be possessive, but can learn that people are no threat. In fact, humans are mighty helpful. Every now and again, take the chewie away from the demo puppy, then dig into pocket or pouch for a tasty treat. Furnish this to the dog and then re-commence assisting him with his chewie.

Emphasize that you did not bribe the dog by showing him the treat up front. It's important that they consistently supply it, but it must always be hidden for these exercises (an emergency is another situation entirely where anything, including bribery, goes). Finish by telling them their goal is for the dog to enjoy their presence around his chew toys and to wag his tail in anticipation of goodies when they are taken away. When coaching the students during the practice period, look for opportunities to reinforce them for adjusting angles and for the correct sequence of remove toy, give treat, give toy back.

Once this has been demonstrated, issue a high-value chewie to all class members for use during explanations and class demos to keep puppies occupied so the humans can attend to the instructor. You can prompt exchanges at regular intervals. Students can also be asked to bring a favorite chew toy from home for this purpose.

Another version of this game involves a Kong™ that is so tightly stuffed the dog is having difficulty extracting the goodies. Sit with the dog and occasionally take the Kong from him in order to extract a good bit with finger or implement. This gets the message across to the dog that humans are (literally) handy to have around one's recalcitrant Kongs.

2. Bowl-bonus game. To prepare for the demo and exercise, put a handful of some relatively unattractive kibble in bowls, one for each puppy and one for the demo dog. In a small ziplock bag, put a few pieces of freeze-dried liver, grilled chicken, or roast beef. Keep the bag sealed and hidden in a bait pouch or pocket. Demo by putting the bowl down and letting a puppy go to town on the kibble. Withdraw to at least six feet, then approach. Once at the puppy, remove the bowl, open your bag, add the tasty bonus to the bowl, and give it back. Be sure to narrate the puppy's point of view for the students: "Okay, she approached and took my bowl away and, wow, did the meal ever get tastier then! I hope she does that again…" Send them off to practice a few reps and look for and point out owners who nail the sequence exactly right.

Ideally, puppy owners should add as many bonuses as possible at home and one way to encourage this is to send students home with a ziplock bag with seven different bonuses in it, one for each day of the coming week. The following week you can check whether anyone noticed any guarding and whether any particular bonuses went over especially well. This helps firm up reinforcer hierarchies, which is helpful for general training.

3. Placement practice. This exercise is good for location guarding prevention—dogs that threaten and defend sofa, bed or other choice sleeping spots. It's good to have a few dog beds and crates in the classroom for students to employ for practice, as well as a sofa, if you can manage it, for those dogs that are allowed on the furniture at home. Demo the following sequence:

1. cue dog onto dog bed ("go to bed")
2. prompt or lure dog on to the bed
3. praise
4. cue dog off bed ("off the bed please")
5. prompt dog off
6. praise and food reward

Repeat the demo, underscoring that you are cuing before prompting so that eventually the dog will anticipate the prompt and start performing for just the cue. Also point out that you are supplying the higher value reward—praise plus food—for getting off, not on. If you have time, an extended demo where you also work in a down-stay, makes a strong impression. As soon as possible, fade out any visible food lures, while still rewarding the dog 100% of the time each time he gets off on cue. An intermittent reinforcement schedule comes much, much later.

I know trainers who make final prioritization decisions in a particular session based on a week one or pre-class owner poll, or even based on the breeds in the class. Breed predispositions and owner preferences allow you to make a more informed choice about which exercises to omit or assign as homework only, which to demo, and which to both demo and allocate a practice and coaching period for.

Fighting Dog Rehabilitation

Dear Jean,

Six months ago I adopted a Pit Bull from a fabulous rescue group. They screen the adopters carefully and all the dogs are thoroughly tested. Abigail is now a year and a half and the sweetest dog I've ever owned. She loves everyone and is excellent with other dogs. The rescue group cautioned me

KEY CONCEPTS
Gameness
Genetic drift
Redirected bites
Hierarchy variables

that she could still become aggressive to other dogs, but that her disposition with people would not change. How can this be? And, if she does become dog aggressive, can training help?

It surely is a sign of a conscientious rescue group that they not only screen dogs and prospective adopters, but fully disclose the warts of the breed they rescue. All breeds have problems and, in the case of Pit Bulls, the ugliest is the potential for "gameness," a strong propensity to fight with other dogs. Whether this genetic predisposition is present in an individual dog can be difficult to predict. This is because of genetic drift in most lines away from the breed's original function. Pit Bulls were originally bred for bull-baiting and dog-fighting around the turn of the last century, and there was strong selection pressure at that time for the suite of characteristics that made a superior specimen: off the charts pugnacity with other dogs, unwillingness to back down in a fight, failure to read appeasement gestures from other dogs admitting defeat, the characteristic body type and, interestingly, a strong inhibition against redirected bites to humans meddling in the fight. This last quality comes as a surprise to many people who have been swayed by the spectacular media coverage of Pit Bull attacks against people. While aggression to other dogs is central to correct breed type, aggression to people is anathema.

In more recent times there has been massive random ("backyard") breeding of Pit Bulls. Once the selection pressure for game characteristics was lifted in favor of size, look, or nothing in particular, the genetic cards were shuffled. So whether some, none, or all of the characteristics of a fighting dog will be present in an individual animal is impossible to tell until the dog is socially mature. This is because there are two onset periods. One is early—often evident while the puppy is still in its litter, relentlessly fighting with siblings in a fashion that is much, much more intense than the play-fighting that all normal puppies engage in.

The second group of game animals present normally as puppies and as young adults. Then, in spite of extensive socialization to other dogs and normal play skills, gameness creeps in sometime between age one and three. This is the reason your rescue group is being prudent about whether your dog is out of the woods with regard to dog-dog aggression. And, as they point out, this quality is completely unrelated to the dog's disposition toward people.

How to rehabilitate game-bred dogs is a fascinating question. It is of course a different question from whether such behavior modification should be attempted. The position of most responsible Pit Bull groups is that dogs with propensities to fight should be tightly managed, i.e., diligently kept away from opportunity. In my opinion, this is the best approach in terms of both safety and efficiency. But rather than explore the ethics or cost-benefit merits of approaching such dogs with behavior modification, I'm going to focus on the technical aspects of a rehabilitation performed by a trainer at The San Francisco SPCA.

The dog in question was an apparent Pit Bull-Chow cross that came into the shelter four years ago. While stellar with people, she attacked any dog within sight and in the relentless fashion characteristic of game dogs. There was no social behavior whatsoever directed at dogs. The choices appeared to be: 1) carefully adopt her out to a remote home with strong admonitions to the adopter about the results of dog encounters; or 2) euthanize her. One of our trainers, Kim Moeller, who had worked on more routine dog-dog aggression problems before, pitched the idea of taking a few months to work on her. The prospect of gaining knowledge—success or no—was too great to pass up, so everyone was supportive of her plan.

A key question when approaching aggression cases of any kind is that of whether the dog is "upset," i.e., whether there is any component of fear, anxiety, or other negative emotion. If the answer is yes, it behooves the trainer to have classical counter-conditioning, the replacement of that emotion with a more favorable one, as part of the agenda. But if the answer is no, straight operant conditioning, the manipulation of consequences contingent on specific target behaviors, is the way to go. Because a plausible case could be made both ways in the case of severe dog-fighting, Kim decided to both build a favorable conditioned emotional response (CER) and employ negative punishment for the worst outbursts of aggression.

Those well acquainted with applied behavior analysis will see a paradox here. The desensitization and counter-conditioning (D&C) procedure, wherein the dog is exposed to stimulus dogs at an intensity that does not elicit aggression and the pairing of the presence of other dogs with gobs of praise and extremely high value food, hinges on the presumption that other dogs are a fear-evoking stimulus. If so, the D&C will make gains. And, if so, any negative punishment, which would be removing her from the situation, should actually function as a negative reinforcer. Removing someone from something that scares them should be a reinforcing event, not a punishing one. And, if it was a punishing event, it is a "liked" stimulus and so there should be no need for D&C!

Interestingly, both techniques seemed to pay dividends: the dog improved. The key desensitization hierarchy variables turned out to be the stimulus dog's novelty to her, the stimulus dog's degree of animation, and how "warmed up" our Pit-Chow was. Until she was very advanced, the first trial of the day was always dicier than mid-session and late in the session trials, independent of the other parameters. And so, early in training, the stimulus dog would be familiar to her and passive. Less familiar dogs and novel dogs were introduced late in the session and the dogs would be passive or kept still.

Gradually, these parameters were edged up independently and, eventually, piled up. Another element that varied was the degree of mechanical control. In early training and at key raises in stimulus intensity, she wore a (pre-desensitized) secure muzzle, a Gentle Leader head collar and was on a six-foot leash. In the earliest sessions, she would charge the stimulus dog at any level of stimulus intensity. Kim's strategy was to physically prevent the attack using these physical controls and then supply the broad praise and food (remember, this is a classical technique—the food is not contingent on her behavior, but rather on the presence of the stimulus dog). Over time, as so often happens in these cases, the presence of the stimulus dog caused her to anticipate the food and orient to the handler from whom the food would be coming, rather than charge the dog. At this point the variables above came into play.

Around this time, time outs were applied for charging. This brings us back to our apparent paradox. Why would removal from the situation be punishing? It is possible that, by this point, the sessions were a welcome diversion to her and a source of praise and treats. Being marched back to her kennel therefore functioned as a strong punisher. It's also possible the kennel was stressful and so an element of positive punishment crept in. And, it's possible that for a fighting dog, being removed from dogs is a punisher and so the technique would have worked well right off the bat. But if this is the case, then D&C should have been ineffective. A possible answer here is that she was being desensitized to attack triggers such as novelty and movement, rather than to dogs as a fear-evoking stimulus per se.

Six months into the training she began playing with other dogs. We were all floored. Her social circle was carefully expanded, the physical controls lifted, and she was adopted out with full disclosure and a lot of post-adoption support. Amazingly, her gains held on follow-up and to this day she regularly attends dog parks without incident.

Predatory Drift

Dear Jean,

Our dog, Henry, killed a dog at the park a month ago. We are still reeling from the shock and I can't begin to imagine how the poor owners of that dog are coping. We have kept him on leash and away from dogs ever since. He is five years old and had gotten along perfectly with other dogs until

KEY CONCEPTS
Predatory drift
Predatory behavior
Social facillitation

this incident. He had several playmates and my sister and dog-sitter both have dogs with which he has co-habited peacefully for weeks at a time. We called a trainer immediately and she explained that this was predatory behavior. This is puzzling to us because all the time we have had Henry he has never been much of a hunter—no chasing after cats, bikes, or cars and an excellent recall on walks in the woods. He is fairly large—65 pounds—and the dog he killed was small—eleven pounds. I can see how this would make it easier for Henry to kill the dog, but not how it would contribute to his wanting to kill this dog as he has interacted peacefully with countless small dogs in his life. Could it still be hunting? Will he ever be trustworthy again?

Given this history, I think this was an example of what Ian Dunbar has coined predatory drift. It's worth summarizing what predation is before examining predatory drift.

Although often lumped under the banner "aggression," predation is food acquisition rather than agonistic (fisticuffs within a species) or defensive behavior, although some of the behaviors in the canine predatory sequence—most notably biting—share some topography with aggression. Predatory behavior warrants careful attention because the results are more often extremely damaging than the results of routine defense and competition.

Some dogs display frank predatory behavior toward other dogs the same way they might toward squirrels, cats, and other critters. Most such dogs direct regular social behavior toward dogs on other occasions or confine their predation to small dogs, or running dogs only. Each dog will have a profile, broad or narrow, of the targeted dogs and contexts that elicit the behavior. There are also key divisions among these dogs regarding which parts of the predatory sequence they are predisposed to. For instance, a dog may be a maniacal chaser but demonstrate great restraint if ever a prey item is caught (a Golden Retriever might gleefully run down a squirrel but have no idea what to do with it once it's caught—the squirrel, is presumably freaked out but unscathed). Others are "finishers," i.e., they finish the predatory sequence by killing what they catch. Terriers are the poster children for this phenomenon although there may be over-representation of other breeds, such as Siberians. As an interesting side note, this incredible genetic elasticity in the dog predatory sequence has allowed for the exaggeration through selective breeding of many of our favorite stylized predation behaviors such as scent-work, pointing, flushing, and herding.

Dogs who are known finishers are best managed (kept away from opportunity). I would also elect to manage dogs that are not known finishers if they target small dogs. This usually manifests when the latter are running or scurrying (retired racer syndrome). The risk of injury is too high, the behavior harder than most to modify, and the management usually easy to implement.

I believe Henry's unfortunate incident was the result of an equally serious, but less well-known phenomenon, predatory drift. Unlike regular predation, which is motivated as such from the get-go, predatory drift is the kicking in of predatory reflexes in an interaction that begins as a social interaction. And, unlike predation, which is predictably elicited in a known quantity by the presence of a member of the target group, predatory drift can occur among dogs who had never been predatory before and may never be again after. It kicks in because of specific contextual triggers. The riskiest contexts are:

- Play or a squabble between two dogs extremely different in size, especially if the smaller dog panics, yelps, and/or struggles. The simulation of a prey item is so convincing that the roles in the interaction drift from a social scuffle to predator-prey. The greater the size disparity, the greater the risk, for three reasons. Firstly, the likelihood of the smaller dog getting inadvertently stepped on or otherwise ouched, even in a normal play session with a reasonably gentle dog, is greater if the dog in question is really tiny. Secondly, I would speculate that the tinier the dog, the better the simulation of a prey item to the bigger dog. Finally, the ease with which the larger dog can grab and shake the smaller one goes up as size difference increases. Grab and shake is often present in predatory drift incidents. Most of us have seen dogs grab and shake toys. Even if non-lethal pressure is exerted, a grab and shake inflicted on a small dog can break its neck.

- Two or more dogs "teaming up" during intense play, or two or more dogs acting together in a chase or squabble context with a dog that begins to panic, yelp, and/or struggle. Dogs have also been known to attack injured dogs and this effect is also facilitated by the attacking unit being two or more dogs as opposed to one.

Because predatory drift can occur in dogs without any particular history, all owners and practitioners should exercise some diligence in the two contexts above—large to small interactions and "double team" (two+ vs. one). While it is quite true that many such interactions are completely benign, predatory drift is common enough that most dog people have either witnessed it or know someone who has. The risks multiply if both factors are present. Another obvious factor that increases risk is the involvement of a known predatory dog in the mix, especially a finisher.

If this rings true for Henry and depending on the recommendations of your trainer, it could be that Henry will be given the green light for continued play and socializing with large dogs, but kept clear of small dogs from now on.

Breed Specific Legislation and Behavior—An Inconvenient Truth?

The other night I was at dinner with a group of dog trainers and the conversation turned to breed specific legislation. Now I must preface what follows with the assurance that these were, without exception, progressive-thinking and enlightened people, many of whom had been in dogs for decades. All deplore hysteria-based, arcane laws

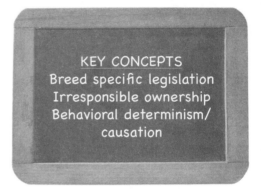

KEY CONCEPTS
Breed specific legislation
Irresponsible ownership
Behavioral determinism/
causation

banning various breeds thought to be over-implicated in serious dog attacks, as have been enacted in numerous jurisdictions.

The question went around the table: if you ruled the world, would you ban any breeds of dog and, if so, which? One might think that a professional and wildly pro-dog crowd such as this would rise above our breed biases and sagely and in unison intone that what we really needed to ban was irresponsible dog ownership. But no. Within two and a half minutes we had (enthusiastically) banned all breeds, with the following exceptions:

Cavalier King Charles Spaniels
Brussels Griffons
Clumber Spaniels
English Cocker Spaniels
Whippets
Norwich and Norfolk terriers
Pugs and French Bulldogs

A couple of lobbying efforts were mounted to get some cherished breeds in under the wire. For instance, someone pointed out that there were no actual big dogs and then opened a negotiation for Newfoundlands. "I'll give you your mini-Aussies, Papillons and Chinese Cresteds if you instate Newfies." "No," a hold-out snapped back. "Newfies will require those plus Standard Poodles. We need a non-shedding, no, the world needs a non-shedding option. We don't need drooling." "Cresteds don't shed. Forget it." And so Newfies were shot down and after more fierce, but feckless bartering and impassioned pitches, the only other breed to squeak in was Italian Greyhounds. The final smug consensus was that we were, in fact, quite generous to give people the choice of ten breeds. On a worse day, it might have ended up All Cavs All The Time. The spike in breaking and entering alone gives one pause. And never mind the Flyball teams.

Interestingly, Pit Bulls were not in the first or even second wave of breeds struck from planet earth. They came in around neck and neck with other medium to large semi-caffeinated breeds. Those genius Border Collies and darling, telegenic Jack Russells were the gold and silver medalists of Let's Never Make Any More (the bronze was a dead heat between Siberian Huskies and Akitas). We culled for high activity level, we culled for anything remotely resembling drivey or compulsive behavior, and we smote all breeds that were suspiciousness of strangers, along with breeds frequently presented with refractory housetraining problems, thus decimating the toys.

I am by no means attempting to tar all dog behavior people with the same brush. We were a small, cynical band of dog eugenicists gleefully banning breeds as dark humor round the table that night, by no means representative of dog people in general. At least I don't think so. I would submit, however, that we overlap with virtually all dog people insofar as we acknowledge that genes affect behavior. This notion is in fact usually a no-brainer for anyone who knows dogs. Ray Coppinger famously pointed out that it would be hard to imagine more divergent MO's than those of flock-guarding breeds like Great Pyrenees and flock-herding dogs like Border Collies. The former protect the flock from predators and the latter move the flock by stalking them, just like predators. No one seriously suggests that this is solely the result of rearing practices.

I admit I find it worrisome, the readiness with which we accept genetic influence on behavior in general, but then flip 180-degrees to a no-genes-ever-ever position when the question of breed specific legislation (BSL) comes up. The only acceptable rallying cry seems to be "it's entirely irresponsible ownership." It is undeniably true that there is no credible evidence demonstrating over-representation of any breeds in egregious aggression incidents. BSL fighters have rightly drawn attention to the poor quality of the research. It is also undeniably true that, as with all behavior, causation is and will always be multi-factorial, i.e., a conspiracy of genes woven together with environment. But what if credible research does come down the pike and what if such evidence concludes that genetics is a factor? Not the only factor, but a factor. What then?

I wonder if part of our gene-o-phobia has to do with assessing blame. For dog lovers and sympathizers, it is easier to place dogs in the role of victim when failures of commission and omission during an otherwise "good" dog's lifetime are at the root of anti-social behavior. However, if it is the dog's "nature"—something in him, something he is born with—he's evil. But wait a minute. The dog is no more in control of the genetic cards he is dealt than he is in control of the owner he is dealt. Sure, it's bad luck to draw an owner that knocks you around, fails to socialize you, fails to train you, but it's no picnic to be saddled with one hundred or more generations of selective breeding to view unfamiliar humans as threatening or be unable to back down from a fight.

If ever evidence comes down—and it's no long shot—that genes influence aggression the way they influence all behavior, we'll have the non dog-loving public to face. "Yeah, sorry, we kind of knew genes mattered in behavior but, hey, the crappy research on dog attacks and blunt instrument of 'breed bans' were sure easy targets." We may get a less than sympathetic ear, too, from owners who knocked themselves out doing everything right with dogs whose genomes imposed a steel ceiling on friendliness to strangers or other dogs. Many, many of these innocent people were not issued much in the way of package warnings by whoever produced their animals and so go on to blame themselves, aided and abetted by our oh-it's-always-rearing anti-BSL war cry.

If it comes down to this, our best shot at protecting breeds from being banned would be to change the genes within breeds, so that they're not at higher risk for aggressive behavior. But you can't change what you don't acknowledge.

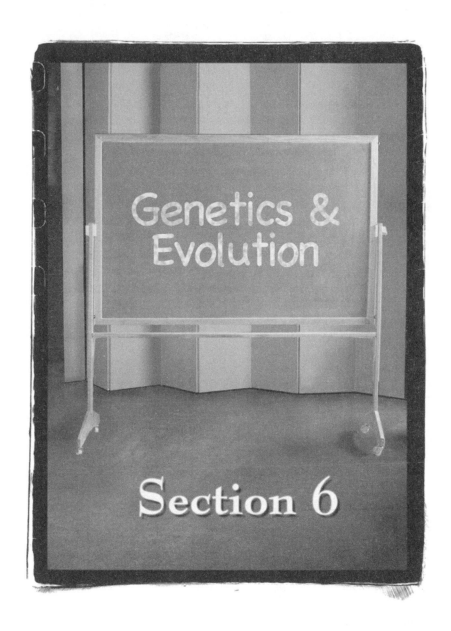

Genetics & Evolution

Section 6

My Genes Made Me Do It

Dear Jean,

*I've had dogs my whole life
and lived through more
behavior problems than I care
to count. In my experience,
putting an outdoor recall on
a Beagle or getting German
Shorthair to relax are rather
like banging one's head against
the wall compared to getting
a Labrador to like people. Is it
worth any time or effort trying to change behavior that is genetic? There
seem to be a lot of opinions out there. Even scientists seem to have no
consensus. What is the current thinking on the nature vs. nurture thing?*

KEY CONCEPTS
Nature vs. nurture
Standard social science
model of behavior
Genetic predisposition

Dog people are no exception when it comes to human fascination with the question of environmental and genetic influences on behavior. The mapping of the human genome and recent celebration of the 50th anniversary of the discovery of the structure of DNA have redoubled interest in genetic influences. Books such as Steven Pinker's *The Blank Slate* make an increasingly strong case for the impact of our genes on everything from what diseases we are likely to get to what kinds of spouses we are likely to marry. Pinker's ideas collide rudely with what he calls the Standard Social Sciences Model (SSSM) of behavior, i.e., the prevailing and politically correct view that we are virtual blank slates and thus products of our culture, upbringing, and environmental influences. What Pinker is urging is for us to rise above what's known as the naturalistic fallacy, the mistaken idea that just because something is a certain way in nature, it is therefore how it ought to be ("natural" = "good"). If genetic influences exist and/or are powerful, then morally legitimizing oppression, discrimination, or other societal ills is the ill-founded fear. He also points out that the monster in the closet for us may not so much be genetic determinism, but determinism period, and that that one is inescapable. Behavior is determined. Often complex, but always determined.

There is actually good consensus among most scientists that there is no "nature-nurture" dichotomy at all. All behavior is the product of a complex interaction between genes and environment. Just as it is meaningless to ask whether a rectangle is a product of its length or its height, it is meaningless to ask whether a certain behavior is a product of genes or the environment. The answer is always both. There is no such thing as one on its own.

Interestingly, in the case of dog people, popular bias has historically swung the other way. Our intimate familiarity with breeds and the behavioral proclivities that stem from their original functions make too strong a case for us to deny genetic influence. Border Collies have more herding "instinct" than Newfoundlands, Pointers are keener bird dogs than Bichons, and Labradors and Goldens are easier to socialize to strangers than Chows and Akitas. The mechanism is said to be genes "for" herding or hunting or suspiciousness of strangers. The reality is that mechanisms are more complex. Genes are simply coded instructions to flip other genes on or off and to manufacture proteins. They are turned on and off during both embryonic development and throughout life. The turning on and off function, interestingly, is not always under control of other genes—it can be triggered by something in the environment. The sex of crocodiles, for example, is determined by nest temperature during the middle trimester of incubation. The genes specify the rules governing sex determination, but the environment actually "chooses" the sex. Labeling such a phenomenon the result of either genes or environment is patently incorrect.

More intriguing wrinkles about genetics and expressed traits were raised a few years ago when scientists at Texas A&M successfully cloned the first cat. One finding was that the cloned cat's coat markings differed significantly from the donor cat. Although the two are genetically identical, differences in the turning on and off of genes during embryological development made for two quite different looking cats. The mind boggles at the possible implications of this for brain development and behavior. And, as though this weren't sufficiently complex, consider the notion that the very environment that many think of as the alternative to "genetic" influence was literally the selector of those genes during the evolutionary history of the animal.

Another interesting notion about mechanisms behind genetically wired behavior was put forward by B.F. Skinner. He hypothesized that what is genetically determined in animals is not necessarily a behavior, but the capacity to be reinforced by a certain kind of event and that this, in turn, impacts behavior. Ducklings are not hard-wired to follow a moving stimulus, he argued, but hard-wired to be reinforced by proximity, which then reinforces the behavior of following. Rabid Skinnerian thinking is strongly out of fashion these days, but many of Skinner's ideas, such as this one, suggest mechanisms to explore in gene-behavior interaction research.

So What About Dogs?
Worries about Pinker's slippery slope of legitimizing something because "it's natural" are also prevalent in dog behavior. For instance, there is little agreement among people in dog behavior and training about whether aggression is normal behavior or some sort of pathology. Part of this debate is driven by a legitimate question—treatment strategies may depend on whether there is disease present—but a larger part is, I think, driven by the is/ought fallacy. For instance, I have personally gone on record as saying that a significant percentage of aggression in dogs is normal behavior. This statement is frequently misinterpreted to mean that I therefore think it's okay for dogs to be aggressive.

The more difficult fallacy to shake is that of the presumed immutability of behavior with a strong genetic component. The bias among most dog people is that behavior with an identifiable predominantly environmental cause is much more plastic (modifiable) than behavior with an identifiable predominantly genetic cause. This intuitive presumption is actually very questionable. There does not seem to be a tidy correlation between how much a behavior is influenced by genetic predisposition and its susceptibility to behavior modification. All kinds of behavior with massive genetic influence—grabbing sandwiches off tables, puppy mouthing, urine marking, intolerance of physical restraint, guarding resources—are routinely modified using standard operant and classical conditioning.

The reason they are modifiable is that the ability to change one's behavior due to environmental contingencies is also hard-wired. The capacity to learn is itself genetic. This undermines to a large degree the "it's genetic" line sometimes uttered when behavior modification reaches a dead-end ("don't bother, it's genetic"). It could absolutely be that genetic constraints have collided with behavior in many cases. My sense, however, is that this platform is defaulted to in cases where justification for giving up is needed in cases that go south. If the owner, dog, and practitioner all need off the hook, genes can provide a convenient explanation. My hope, however, is that as understanding of the genetics-behavior connection and behavior mod techniques both improve, this line will need to be trotted out less. There may even emerge tactical insights to speed my Chow up at Flyball.

Genes and Behavior

Dear Jean,

When behavior is hard-wired rather than learned, does it mean it is 100% genetic? How do genes create behavior? Can a single gene influence behavior? How can we be sure it's not environment that's causing changes in behavior that are deemed genetic?

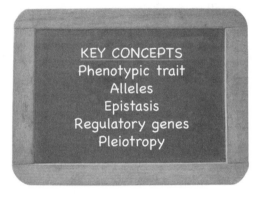

KEY CONCEPTS
Phenotypic trait
Alleles
Epistasis
Regulatory genes
Pleiotropy

These are superb questions. First, it's important to understand that genes can't "make" behavior, especially complex behavior, any more than a single engine part "makes" a car (though a malfunction of a gene can derail behavior just as a faulty engine part can cause a car to break down). Behavior is a phenotypic trait, i.e., it is an observable characteristic of an animal. A phenotypic trait—including "hardwired" or unlearned behavior—is always the end product of an interaction between the animal's genes and the animal's environment. An animal's genotype is the collection of all its genes, whether they are expressed ("visible") in the phenotype or not. How genes do their part starts with the exact spot on the chromosome, called a locus, where the gene resides. Two alleles, which are versions of each gene donated by each parent, are at every locus. The relationship between the two alleles may be additive, which means the phenotype is intermediate between the two. As a hypothetical example, imagine breeding a dog with high drive for toys to a dog with low drive and the offspring are moderately drivey for toys.

The relationship between alleles can also be dominant-recessive to varying degrees, where one allele is expressed in the phenotype and the other, though present and transmissible to offspring, is nearly or completely silent. This is the Mendelian inheritance taught in many biology classes, with eye-color in humans the classic example. To answer your question about whether single genes can influence behavior, the answer is "yes," with the operative word being "influence." Complex traits, such as behavior, are better understood as the product of the actions and interactions of many, many genes. Such traits are called polygenic, which means each individual gene makes up only a small part of the genetic contribution to the trait. Body size is a well-known polygenic trait. Polygenic traits can be additive, as in body size or they can be epistatic, where the product is not intermediate between the genes involved, but rather is more analogous to the dominant-recessive relationship that exists at individual loci. Coat color heredity in many breeds of dog is a familiar example of a phenotypic trait that is governed by epistasis.

Remember, it's far from over once a set of genes are turned on or off. Genes interact with the environment to result in the final phenotypic product, the body part or behavior that we can see. Even body size, though largely polygenically determined, is somewhat influenced by environmental influences like nutrition, illness, etc. In the case of behavior, environmental interactions often play a larger role. For example, famous research on mice bred for high aptitude at running mazes—maze bright mice—and mice bred for low aptitude—maze dull mice—also found that rearing the maze dull mice in a more complex and stimulating environment compensated for their maze dull genes and they performed as well on mazes as maze bright mice.

Environment not only interacts with genes, but can directly affect their activity—it can literally turn them on and off! In fact, about 95% of genes that code at all don't code for proteins on the road to phenotypic traits, but rather regulate the action of other genes. Most of these regulatory genes respond to environmental triggers, which prompt them to turn the protein coding genes on and off, both in utero when the organism is being built, during post-natal development, and right on into adulthood. In other words, genes don't provide recipes in stone on how to build bodies and behave to organisms so much as they participate in a give-and-take process with environmental signals throughout life.

Regulator genes may very well send instructions to genes that are themselves regulator genes. Eventually, further downstream, genes are turned on that will build proteins, specifically enzymes. Enzymes then affect cellular metabolism, which in turn affects other cells. At the end of this chain reaction comes the tiny chemical increments that make up the genetic part of the genetics-environment cocktail that is behavior.

An interesting result of this string of events, all kicked off by a particular regulator gene, is that a single gene can have two or more—sometimes many more—effects! This is called pleiotropy and is quite different from polygenic effects, where multiple genes contribute to one effect. A famous example of pleiotropy occurred during the Russian fox domestication experiment where strong selection for reduced flight distance also produced floppy ears, curled tails, shorter muzzles, and occasionally, even white markings on the coat.

There are different flavors of pleiotropy. For instance, one regulator gene can kick off chain reactions in multiple metabolic pathways in different body systems. Pleiotropy can also occur if a gene sits right next door to another unrelated gene on a chromosome and then both stick together when cut and pasted into the new generation.

So how do we know its genes? The way genes influence behavior can be teased out of the gene-environment interaction in a variety of ways. Even before the advent of molecular genetics, animals with identical or near-identical genotypes were studied in different environments, and animals with different genotypes were studied in identical or near-identical environments. These measures did a reasonable job of controlling for environmental effects. The serendipitous (for science) "experiment" of comparing human identical twins separated at birth yielded revealing data about the effect of genes on behavior.

Direct study of the presence or absence of specific genes and how this impacts behavior is now possible too. Because it is so unlikely that single genes will be found that have profound behavioral effects, researchers concentrate their search for sets of genes that each make their small contribution to a certain behavior. Also, most behavior traits are distributed in a continuous rather than "digital" fashion, which strongly implies multiple genes. For example there isn't an on-off switch for "anxiety" that effectively divides dogdom into dogs completely without a predisposition and those completely riddled.

Research that attempts to link the presence of gene suites with elevated occurrence of certain traits in families can be confounded by partial dominance effects and the fact that the same traits may be brought about by different genetic routes. Scans of full genomes can narrow the search if there is a marker residing in close proximity to a candidate gene that is suspected to be associated with a certain trait. The spot on the genome of a control group without the trait is then compared to the same spot on the genome of the group with the trait.

Experiments can really ice the cake when it comes to nailing down which genes do what. For example, once a suspect gene has been identified, it can be "knocked out" of the genome of mice with genomes that are otherwise identical to a control group of mice and then the two groups compared in minute detail. Transgenics, where genes from another animal, such as a human, are spliced in to an experimental animal is also a fruitful way to directly observe the effects of genes on behavior, body type, and body function. When all these methods converge on the same conclusion, the evidence for the effects of certain genes is extremely compelling.

Adaptive Significance of Various Dog Behaviors

Dear Jean,

I'm reading a book on dog behavior that says the reason dogs chew is to keep their teeth clean and their jaws strong. I'm having some difficulty fully buying this. In my thirty years in dogs, I've had dogs taken to the vet for ingested chew toys and even one broken tooth, and I must say, many, many a middle-aged and older dog for tooth cleaning in spite of plenty of chewing all their lives. My overwhelming impression is that they simply enjoy chewing. Isn't that a more obvious explanation? (P.S. If keeping their teeth clean was such an overriding priority, you'd think they'd like the toothbrush more.)

KEY CONCEPTS
Immediate or proximate causation
Adaptive significance
Selfish genes
Inclusive fitness

Both you and the author of your book may be correct. There are two kinds of answer to "why does he do that?" questions. One kind, called "immediate" or "proximate" causation, involves the hormonal, neurochemical, and sensory precursors and consequences of behavior, such as "enjoying" something. The other kind, called adaptive significance, involves the advantage provided by such hormones, neurochemistry, and sensory apparatus in the environment the animal evolved in. Your or my dog might enjoy chewing, but why does she enjoy it? And why doesn't she "enjoy" 120-degree heat? These ultimate answers are always some variation on the theme, "because they contributed to the fitness of the animal in the environment it evolved in." And so, chewing serves some adaptive function in dogs. Finding high heat aversive and thus avoiding it was also selected for.

When animals behave, they are not driven or triggered in a conscious way by the evolutionary advantage of their behavior, but by the various mechanisms that evolved to serve that end. During evolution, brains that happened to reward dogs when they chewed helped the bodies they were in have slightly better teeth than bodies with brains that didn't happen to reward them when they chewed. The chewing dogs didn't consider or celebrate their slight reproductive advantage. They were busy being rewarded by their brains for chewing. (Incidentally, those same brains evolved mechanisms to respond to environmental contingencies in a flexible way, which we call learning, and you could exploit this module to condition your dogs to like that toothbrush more.)

Let's look at a couple of examples from other species. When male elephant seals duke it out over breeding rights, they aren't calculating the odds of getting their genes into the next generation if they win a sufficiency of such battles any more than their gigantic bodies are conniving to put on as much as weight as possible to achieve the same end. They "feel aggressive" when other males approach their harems and have an irresistible urge to posture and fight. Male elephant seals who don't feel such urges don't contribute their pacifist genes to future generations.

When ducklings follow their mothers around ("imprinting") they are not deducing "I will stay close to my parent to reduce my chances of being preyed upon, ergot improving my chances of surviving and reproducing," but rather running a program that rewards their brains for proximity to large moving objects, and punishes them with anxiety for lack of proximity. Voila, out pops following.

So, if adaptive significance is about the survival of the fittest, the next question becomes, "the fittest what?" Is it the elephant seals vs. the fish they eat? Ducks vs. foxes? Ducks vs. geese? This variety of duck vs. that one? Elephant seals vs. gray seals? This harem vs. that one? This male vs. that one? All these anatomical, physiological, and behavioral adaptations are for the good of something? What's the unit? The answer is that the unit in natural selection is the gene!

Selfish Genes and Altruistic Acts

We've all heard the phrase "good of the species" in wildlife documentary narrations. It appeals to human intuition, but is it correct? Consider an animal whose genes tell him to do some behavior for the "good of the species," let's say throwing himself off a cliff if food supplies are poor one year so that there is more to go around for the rest of his species. Compare him with an individual in the same species whose genes tell him not to throw himself off a cliff, but to eke out as best he can and do his utmost to reproduce. Note that the throw-oneself-off-a-cliff gene does not get passed on whereas the hang-in-there-while-someone-else-throws-themselves-off-a-cliff gene proliferates. Soon the population is filled with non-suicidals.

Then, what about cats going into burning buildings? How is this benefiting the selfish genes of the cat? The answer lies in the concept of inclusive fitness—the sharing of genes between related animals. Genes do exist for altruistic acts—acts directed at saving copies of the same gene housed in another individual. The degree of genetic relatedness dictates the likelihood and intensity of altruistic acts across all species. The cat going into the burning building is saving her kittens, in whose bodies are copies of the very genes that are telling her to do this. They are saving themselves.

In the words of ethologist Richard Dawkins, organisms are survival machines built by genes to move themselves through time. If you give up your own life to save two offspring (each of whom share, on average, 50% of your genes), eight cousins, or your own identical twin, it's a wash from the genes' point of view. If you remain alive while saving them, the gene team is ahead. Of course no one considers these things when they do heroic acts. The mechanisms built by genes to serve this end are bonding, love, and the stuff of which great movies are made.

These same altruistic mechanisms can misfire. I would likely go into a burning building to save my spayed Chow. This is rather bogglingly poor use of parenting resources on many levels. And Lassie got Timmy out from under the tractor. These kinds of fascinating examples notwithstanding, during evolution, the kin selection shotgun got it right enough of the time for the capacity to bond to those around us to have been strongly selected for.

All of this becomes even more wrinkly when we consider a domesticated species like dogs, where we humans are, in many instances, selecting mates and, when the animals will not breed, facilitating this with everything from holding bitches still to artificial insemination. We also intervene in the pregnancy, delivery, and rearing, especially when these go awry. Because of this, some of the mechanisms that evolved in the original evolutionary environment that produced the wild precursors of dogs may be muddled up. The selection pressures are now quite different.

Such interventions by humans are sometimes criticized as meddling with nature and creating non-viable animals. But this overlooks a most interesting point, which is that genes don't care whether they are making it to the next generation by virtue of being in an organism that maximizes its fitness with adaptations that put it on the cover of a David Attenborough video or in an organism that makes a living releasing care-giving behavior in humans (or herding their sheep, or guarding their property).

So, although packs of Pugs would not do well on the open plains, Pugs are enormously more successful than, say, African Wild Dogs, a species beautifully adapted to life on the open plains, but that has dwindled down to 5,000 individuals. Pugs number far more than 5,000 by having enlisted the care and support of humans. So, if you're a gene, you're likely better off, in terms of your long-term immortality, being the gene for brachycephalism in Pugs than for longer running legs in African Wild Dogs.

Want to know more? For information on selfish gene theory and the evolution of bonding and altruism try: Richard Dawkins' *The Selfish Gene*, Matt Ridley's *The Origins of Virtue* and Robert Wright's *The Moral Animal*. If you'd like to find out about or contribute to conservation efforts for African Wild Dogs, visit The African Wild Dog Project at www.africanwilddog.org or via snail mail c/o JN Allen, PhD, DVM, 3618 39th Ave West, Seattle, WA 98199.

Chows vs. Border Collies

Dear Jean,

I was a long-time Pug person until recently when I got a Jack Russell to do agility, and then rescued another one. I feel like I've been relocated to a different planet. I therefore chuckled when I heard you got a Chow. Operant condition your way out of that one (ha ha ha!!). So, what's with the Chow, seriously?

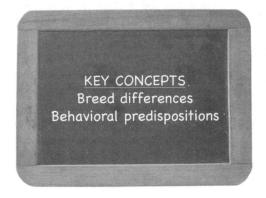

KEY CONCEPTS
Breed differences
Behavioral predispositions

Having been a Border Collie owner since 1980s, I marvel almost daily at my Chow. And at Chows in general. I have gotten into Chows. With the zeal unique to recent breed converts, I foster Chows (www.obeybuffy.org), chat with Chow people on the internet between surfing Chow sites, am riveted to the Chow ring at Westminster, and buy endless Chow shot glasses, nightgowns, and notepaper. I have purchased grooming gear and accessories to the tune of the gross domestic product of a small nation.

Breed differences are the fuel that drives the dog fancy. We are most familiar with conformation standards, but brains are also amenable to artificial selection. Amid behavioral overlap—generic basics such as bonding to owner, use of nose as primary information-gathering tool, propensity to scavenge, and tail wagging—is a rich stream of differences in the tendencies of breeds, both profound and quirky.

Take Border Collies and Chows. Though both bark at the doorbell, the Border Collie spends non-doorbell downtime presenting stuffed Mr. Iguana and watching for flinches away from computer and toward Frisbee™ area. The Chow spends non-doorbell downtime patrolling the yard perimeter and stationing herself at strategically advantageous positions in the house in case the doorbell might ring or, best-case scenario, the Bad Guys enter without ringing.

Both enjoy tug, but the Border Collie plays earnestly and works very, very hard. The Border Collie works very, very hard at everything as a matter of fact. There is a compulsive edge to their favorite activities. Border Collies seem to not so much enjoy activities as relieve mental pressure with them. The Chow is less serious about tug. She holds on, grinning while the other dog (or human) punches itself out dragging her dead weight around in frog position. They both love car rides, but the Border Collie is wound up about the destination, whereas the Chow enjoys the ride.

The Chow is finally starting—after a year of diligent human effort—to chase and catch the odd Frisbee, but in a jaunty, un-earnest way. Her early triumphs consisted of opening her mouth while plopped in the grass, the Frisbee sailing over or bouncing off her well-padded head. She also does Flyball, but the trainers are frowny about the opposite speed issue of most Flyball dogs: rather than requiring hot predatory ritual to motivate her to come back at maximum warp post-box climax, Buffy saunters down, but then kicks it back for the roast beef and gorgonzola. I am thrilled each and every time she does a run, however much it reeks of back-chaining. By contrast, I distinctly remember some genuine angst many years ago when a Border Collie puppy I had was not showing a crazed natural retrieve at age ten weeks. And there is no shortage of Border Collies irritated by food waved at them when they're working on an important task such as moving farm animals around or playing fetch.

With Chows there is not the gift of obedience, but rather a painstakingly orchestrated alignment of obedience behaviors with current Chow life objectives. Set up the right flow chart and they'll do it. Miss a chunk of the flow chart and they don't.

Ray Coppinger points out the wild disparity between the behavioral predispositions of herding dogs and flock guarding dogs, one preying in stylized fashion on stock and the other defending the same stock against predators. There is a certain facility to "training" Pointers to point or "training" Border Collies to herd as so many individuals in these breeds not only find the behaviors enormously self-reinforcing, but do them with the particular style that their lines have been bred for. Rather than shaping behavior by selecting it in real time with reinforcers and punishers, breeding shapes behavior over generations by selecting (reinforcing) and culling (uh, punishing) genes. Subsequent tweaking of performance is then most efficiently obtained by allowing these self-reinforcing activities to continue when the animal is performing as desired or cutting off opportunities to continue contingent on undesired aspects. It's hard-wiring and operant conditioning rolled elegantly into one.

When it comes to behavior modification or training of tasks that are not heavily weighted toward a specialized breed (such as herding, pointing or going to ground), however, the playing field becomes more level. All breeds are endowed with that most interesting adaptation, plasticity, which allows changes to one's behavior based on environmental contingencies encountered during the course of an individual's lifetime. The adding of sits, downs, and heeling on cue, and the removal of jumping up, pulling on leash, guarding bones, and urinating on carpets rely on laws of learning that are universal to vertebrates (and the many invertebrates that have been examined). Where breed comes into play here is in selection of reinforcers and style of performance. Keen trainers are drawn to high-drive dogs, who can be motivated to perform in intense and highly animated fashion by prey-type reinforcers like balls and tug toys. These same dogs tend to do poorly in pet homes where the same unexploited and unchanneled drive translates into chaos and mayhem.

Historically, breed did make a greater difference in obedience training due to traditional training methods that relied heavily on the use of aversive motivators. Whereas some breeds tend to respond to aversives appeasingly, which does not hamper and, arguably, helps the training process, others have a fight/flight/freeze default that can derail training altogether.

Another significant difference between breeds of dog seems to be the ease with which they can be socialized to people. Though all dogs become relaxed and affiliative with family members and people they see often enough, comfort around unfamiliar people varies significantly from dog to dog and trends between breeds seem apparent. Clues to possible mechanisms behind this can be gleaned by domestication experiments, such as the one carried out by geneticist Dimitri Belyaev. Belyaev has become famous for selectively breeding tameness in foxes, animals that in close captivity might break teeth or die from exhaustion attempting to escape their cages, engage in stereotypies, and be incredibly fearful and aggressive around humans. By starting out selectively breeding those animals that fled last when approached, and later selecting for friendliness to people, Belyaev achieved remarkably tame, handleable, pro-social foxes in less than twenty generations. Interestingly, he also obtained piebald coats, floppy ears, curly tails, shorter muzzles, rounded skulls, and barking, which had not been selected for.

Piebald coat color is a common theme in many domesticated species, but does not occur in their wild counterparts. Belyaev has hypothesized that production of L-dopa, a melanin (pigment) precursor, was delayed during development, resulting in white patches on the animal's coat. L-dopa is also an adrenalin precursor, so it's possible that there is lower adrenalin in these animals, which then attenuates fight or flight responses. Serotonin—low levels of which are implicated in anxiety, fear, aggression, depression, and poor impulse control—was significantly higher and corticosteroid levels (stress hormones) lower in the selectively bred foxes. And, the fear period in their development commenced weeks later than that of the wild controls. By breeding for a different neurochemical profile (i.e., tame behavior), Belyaev may have modified genes that control the turning on and off of other key genes for behavior and morphology during the foxes' embryological and post-natal development, such as those that resulted in the pedomorphic (short muzzles, etc.) features.

It's impossible to resist speculating about genetic predispositions to neurochemistry that potentiates higher degrees of fear and aggression in dogs. Even if selective breeding for super ease of socialization never catches on in the dog fancy, this in no way condemns any dog to a lifetime of fight or flight to innocuous stimuli. Our understanding of serotonin modulation by way of everything from exercise, supplements, and nutrition to ever smarter generations of medications increases yearly and this knowledge has already begun to reach dog owners and professionals. My hope is that one day, a sophisticated combination of diligent breeding, mod, and meds will relegate these most serious of behavior problems to history.

Theories of Domestication

Dear Jean,

Are dogs descended from wolves, jackals, or both? When were they domesticated and who did it? Every time I read something on this, they've changed their minds.

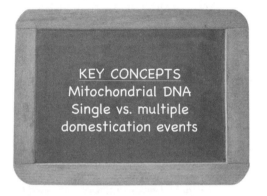

KEY CONCEPTS
Mitochondrial DNA
Single vs. multiple
domestication events

One of the great—but annoying and confusing—things about science is that all conclusions are tentative and as evidence is generated, prevailing theories are morphed or dropped. A great example of this is the hunt for domestic dog origins. It's been a bit of a jigsaw puzzle because the puzzle pieces have come in gradually—research has proceeded at a trickle rather than a flood. And, the puzzle pieces have been made up of evidence from multiple sources: archeological evidence (fossils, bones, artifacts, art), morphological evidence (comparing dog anatomy and physiology to that of wolves), and genetic evidence. For a time, it seemed these sources pointed to different answers, but newer research is filling gaps and pointing to a possible convergence of evidence into one theory.

First of all, the easy part: dogs are descended from gray wolves, not jackals and not coyotes. To understand some of the strongest evidence for this statement, it's necessary to first understand mitochondrial DNA. We're all familiar with the DNA contained in the nucleus of our cells: it contains the recipes for building the proteins that determine most of our genetic traits such as having two legs, two arms, five fingers, straight hair, and a pre-disposition to like asparagus. We each inherit half of our complement of nuclear DNA from each of our parents.

There is another kind of DNA housed in mitochondria, structures that are in our cells, but outside the nucleus. They are mainly involved in energy production for the cell. The reason mitochondria have their own DNA is that they are likely the descendents of nucleus-free cellular organisms that fused with the ancestors of our nucleus-containing cells to make the cells that now make up most of our bodies. Teaming up as a cell within a cell was a win-win situation (symbiosis) for both parties, evolutionarily speaking. Mitochondrial DNA comes in shorter strands than nuclear DNA and is inherited only in the maternal line (everyone, both male and female, gets theirs from their mothers—sperm have insufficient luggage space). It is important because some of it is expressed in our bodies (e.g., cytochrome b mutations that result in decreased exercise tolerance), and also because it has a slow mutation rate, which allows relatively accurate relatedness comparisons across large numbers of generations.

Mitochondrial DNA sequencing has eliminated all discussion about the relationship between dogs, wolves, and coyotes. For example, wolves differ from dogs by less than 0.2% in their mitochondrial DNA whereas they differ from coyotes by approximately 4%. Dogs and wolves are incredibly closely related. In fact, they are literally one species, dogs being a sub-species or variety of wolf. (The definition of a "species" is that all members can inter-breed and produce fertile offspring.)

As for the origins of domestication, the earliest archeological find believed to be a dog dates from 14,000 years ago: a jawbone found in Germany. Smallish dog bones found in the Middle East have been dated at 12,000 years ago. Other archeological finds from this time are more ambiguous: possibly dogs, but also possibly smallish wolves. In Utah, clear evidence of dogs has been dated at approximately 9,000 to 10,000 years ago. This and existing mitochondrial DNA evidence from the mid 1990s initially suggested multiple domestication events in the old and new world. This means that the theory, until very recently, was that different sub-populations of wolf were independently domesticated to produce different ancestral strains accounting for clusters of modern dog breeds.

Then, in 1997, a bombshell paper: mitochondrial DNA evidence collected from a large sample of dogs and wolves prompted the authors to propose a split-off of dogs from wolves over 100,000 years ago. This is an order of magnitude away from the archeological evidence. To explain the discrepancy, it was hypothesized that although this genetic split had taken place, there was insufficient change in body type—especially those hard structures that fossilize more readily—to create any evidence of the split in the fossil record. The 100,000 years ago domestication bombshell later fizzled out due to lack of corroborating evidence. There was more than one way to interpret those results, one of which supported the more recent domestication.

In 2002, two teams of researchers published research converging back on a single domestication event on the order of 15,000 years ago. One team focused on the locale of early domestication, concluding that East Asia is where wolves were first turned into dogs. There were five definite lines, each derived from a single female wolf, with hints of a possible sixth line, all based on extensive mitochondrial DNA analysis. This suggests that dogs caught on like wildfire, spreading to all corners of the globe with human migration.

The other team also provided strong refutation of the multiple domestication events hypothesis by comparing mitochondrial DNA from late Pleistocene dogs from the Old and New Worlds with that of modern dogs. They concluded that all dogs descend from Old World gray wolves and split off from them about 15,000 years ago.

While a formidable tool for researchers into domestication, the slow mutation rate of mitochondrial DNA turns out to be a disadvantage for elucidating the genetic relatedness of modern dog breeds as these have existed for just a few hundred years in the vast majority of cases. So, nuclear DNA evidence was used by researchers who in 2004 published findings that compare the genetics of eighty-five breeds of dog as well as the order of their splitting off from wolves.

In the vast majority of cases, it was possible to correctly identify what breed an individual DNA sample was from. This is testimony to the careful maintenance of separate gene pools within dog breeds.

The earliest split-off from wolves was a branch consisting of Shar Peis, Shiba Inus, Chows and Akitas. Next came Basenjis. The third branch was made up of Alaskan Malamutes and Siberian Huskies (which, incidentally, were difficult to distinguish genetically). The fourth group to split off were Afghans and Salukis. Then came a giant group with the most modern origins, consisting of all the other breeds that were analyzed. Interestingly, Pharaoh and Ibizan Hounds, considered extremely old breeds, were in the modern-origins group genetically. What this means is that modern Pharaoh and Ibizan Hounds are re-creations of the dogs drawn on interior walls in ancient Egypt.

Breeder Power

A few years ago I had the opportunity to tour a guide dog facility and chat with the behavior staff there. The organization employs primarily dogs from their own breeding program with unflappable, friendly dispositions high on the breeding criteria list along with good health and aptitude for their work. After puppies are

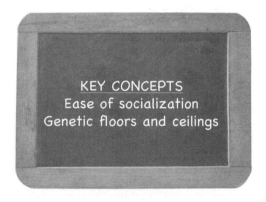

KEY CONCEPTS
Ease of socialization
Genetic floors and ceilings

weaned, they are sent to puppy raisers for the first year before being trained and placed. The puppy raiser is given a credential and vest that allows the puppy into public places for the purpose of extensive socialization.

While we toured the campus, the head of training told me a story of one puppy that was given to first-time puppy raisers who proceeded to drop the ball. Complete non-compliance. An adult man and woman with no children lived in a rural spot with no neighbors for miles. Not only did they fail to get the puppy into busses, restaurants, and shopping malls, onto busy streets and playgrounds full of children, they failed to get the puppy out. At all. The puppy never left the farm. For the entire first year of its life. And there were no visitors. Zero.

My eyes bugged out when I heard this and I expected to then get a sad tale of a skittish adult, shy around new people, and anxious about new places, sights, and sounds. Not a candidate for training and likely a difficult placement as a pet. Instead the trainer brightly informed me that the dog, on initial testing, had been a little more reactive to sudden noises than average but, otherwise, was normal: gregarious and unruffled. More amazingly, the trainer was not at all surprised by this outcome, explaining that extensive socialization is, for them, a redundant line of defense rather than a compensation for wobbly genetics.

This is a terrific example of the most useful way to think about the interaction between genetics (nature) and environment (nurture). Imagine a continuum for a behavior trait, such as neophobia (fear of novelty—notably being non-gregarious or uncomfortable around unfamiliar people). We could name the continuum "Ease of Socialization." At the far right is complete friendliness with new people. At the other end is complete distrust and spookiness with new people. The phenotypes of all dogs could be placed along this continuum at a specific point that represents how sociable they are with unfamiliar people. This phenotype—the actual behavior we can see and measure in the real world—is derived from the placement on the continuum of dog's genetic "envelope" together with the exact spot in that envelope, which depends on environment (most notably early environment).

For example, in the diagram is a dog at mid-point on the continuum. The dog is not as spooky as a fox, but the owner would like him to be better with strangers. If the owner were to ask "can he be made better?" the only honest answer would be "I don't know." We don't know because the genetic envelope—the "floor" and "ceiling"—is usually not known. It could be the black envelope, with the dog already at the genetic "ceiling" or it could be the grey envelope, showing significant room for improvement with well-executed behavior modification, or another envelope. The dog at the guide dog organization had a narrow envelope well at the right hand end of the scale.

Ease of Socialization

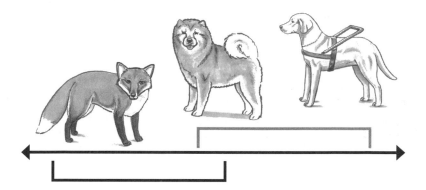

We live in a society with a strong "nurture" bias. A child can be molded into anything with the right upbringing and anyone can grow up to be president. Most of us in the dog world oppose deplorable measures such as breed-specific legislation (BSL) and insurance biases against breeds (rightfully, in my opinion—there has not been any convincing evidence that breed specific legislation does anything to curtail dog related injuries or fatalities).

I submit that there is a bit of an uncomfortable truth we have yet to fully face. And that is that there is some deliberate breeding of dogs with not only low-ish floors on important traits such as ease of socialization, but low-ish ceilings as well. A low ceiling means that even if environmental intervention—socialization, health care, training etc.—is maxed out, the dog will only get X friendly to strangers. And sometimes X isn't very friendly.

If you read through breed standards you'll occasionally see euphemisms for difficult-to-socialize. "Aloof and reserved with strangers," and "observant and vigilant with strangers" mean exactly this. There is no question that dog fanciers cherish the notion that "correct" temperament in some breeds is less than gregarious with unfamiliar people. If the dogs in question are being employed in their original function of personal or property guardian, then the argument could absolutely be made that it is a responsible breeding practice. If the dogs in question are primarily ending up pets, it's much more difficult to defend. If it ends up providing ammunition for those that would ban breeds or reduce the privileges of dogs in our society, then we all hold a stake.

There is a market out there for dogs who can tell the good guys from the bad guys, allowing the former every liberty, while biting the latter. It's a notion out of 1960's television. The problem is dogs don't have radar for good people and bad people. For every dog that makes headlines as a hero for nailing a would-be burglar or attacker are likely hundreds of other dogs who bit the gardener, visitor, or approaching child for exactly the same reasons: being not fully comfortable about strangers.

Any coveting of low ease of socialization in dogs that are expected to be someone's pet is a virtual make-work program for trainers and behaviorists who counsel on fear and aggression to strangers cases. Too often not only did the owner do all the right things vis-a-vis early environment, socialization, and training, they threw every available resource at healing the dog, who has collided with a low genetic ceiling. In some cases prospective buyers didn't read through the euphemisms when they did their breed homework and then were not provided with frank "package warnings" from their breeder. In other cases, the owners thought that's what they wanted or thought they could compensate (or were told they could compensate) with diligent early intervention. It is not only heartbreaking for these individual families but, in the current BSL-crazy climate, a bad advertisement for dogs in general.

Geneticists and informed breeders know that you can't have it all. We may want to consider whether it's worth having "reserved," "discerning," and "one-family" seventy-five pound dogs around as accurate historical artifacts when a good many such animals are destined to end up as family pets.

Dog Moms and Other Evolutionary Misfires

Dear Jean,

Years ago I remember you poking fun during a seminar at dog people who had purchased vehicles to accommodate their dogs. I just heard you bought an SUV for yours. Backatcha!

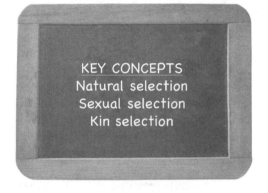

KEY CONCEPTS
Natural selection
Sexual selection
Kin selection

Yes, and with a coordinating interior color! I bet, too, that many of those holding this book have dog vehicles, put dog-friendliness and practicality high on the list when purchasing or renting housing, expend some serious time each day to dog care and dog activities, frown over the latest dog nutrition articles, sign petitions for dogs, and give time and money to dog charities. We are the Dog Moms (and Dads).

Dogs Moms buying SUV's for dogs is, to me, one of the most interesting topics in all of behavior, encompassing love, sex, the struggle for survival and, of course, the human-animal bond. Let's begin at the beginning. Everything we are and everything we do—our behavior—has one ultimate aim, which is the transportation of genetic information through time. Every living organism alive is the culmination of an unbroken string of successful reproducers. We see, think, cooperate, wage war, and enjoy cheesecake all because teams of genes that produced these traits out-reproduced teams of genes that did not in our evolutionary history.

Evolution is governed by two forces, natural selection and sexual selection. Natural selection refers to differential survival under the environmental pressures that face living things: getting enough food, not becoming injured or ill, avoiding becoming food, coping with climate ups and downs, basically surviving long enough to reproduce. Sexual selection is a different pressure. Survival is great, but what if you don't breed? All those good genes that helped you survive don't get passed on. So, you also have to win at the mating game. To do this, another suite of characteristics may be needed.

Mates—and we're usually talking females, who build larger sex cells, then endure pregnancy and nursing, and so have the bigger investment—would like to combine their genes with the best quality genes out there. So how does a girl know? The answer is warfare and advertising. Males must out-compete other males on a variety of battlefields, which can result in arms races of body size and weaponry, and they dazzle females with outlandishly expensive displays, plumage, gifts, nests, and the like, all saying, in effect, "I am so incredibly fit and can so easily throw off parasites and all that so I can afford to prance/grow/build this outraaaaageous thing. I will give you babies that are stupendous and attractive like me."

Here's the most interesting part. Although I use the image of some male surviving, fighting, and advertising in order to reproduce, the unit "trying" to get passed on is not the organism himself (or herself). The units of natural and sexual selection are the individual genes in that organism. The organism is a vehicle that teams of genes build to transport themselves through time. There are genes that code for basic proteins common to all life that have achieved immortality over literally billions of years. That's success.

The idea of genes as the units of selection represented a paradigm shift in biology away from "group selection," the notion that animals behave for the "good of the group." And, when biologists say that genes are "selfish," it simply means they don't care whether the organism lives or dies a Braveheart death, as long as they make it to the next generation. As it happens, a good many traits that are in the genes' interest are in the interests of the organism. There is some use of metaphor here. Genes aren't trying to do anything. They don't sit around thinking about their "interests." The ones that happen to team up with other genes and produce traits that happen to enhance the survival and reproduction of their vehicles proliferate. Actually, plenty of crafty, but naughty, genes hitch rides through the generations not by enhancing survival and reproduction of their vehicles; so-called "junk DNA" codes for nothing except "copy me."

When it came along, selfish gene theory tied the fields of evolutionary biology and genetics together beautifully, but there was a snag. The snag was altruistic behavior. Why on earth would selfish genes code for their vehicle to make any kind of sacrifice? Enter W.D. Hamilton. In the early 1960's, Hamilton came up with mathematical formulas to support the idea of inclusive fitness, i.e., kin selection. His theories allowed testable predictions, which were born out. Genes don't care about which vehicle they move through time in, so altruistic behavior between animals that share genes is in proportion to their genetic relatedness.

Which brings us to the strong bond between parent and offspring. There is little that is more in the interest of genes than coding for traits that help them move successfully down generations, i.e., competent parenting. Genes that coded for Deadbeat Parents were out-reproduced by The Nurturers. The mechanism for recognizing kin and then directing altruistic behavior at them is not some artful measuring of degree of relatedness. It is very likely mediated neurochemically and hormonally (in humans at least—insects very often use scent).

So, it could be that when Dog Moms nurture and spend time with their dogs, they experience the same suite of brain chemicals—some combination of oxytocin, vasopressin, dopamine, serotonin, and norepinephrine—that mothers experience when nurturing their babies. If this is so, a Dog Mom's body can't compute the societal chant of "it's just a dog" because it is responding via machinery that evolved to respond to offspring. You may know (or may yourself be) someone who responds more strongly to puppies than to babies. Directing parenting resources at puppies is a colossal misfire, from your genes' point of view. They are at a dead end if a Dog Mom doesn't have any human children.

Which begs the question: how are Dog Moms made? What causes neurochemistry that makes dogs the target of parenting behavior? Exclusive (i.e., dogs instead of, rather than in addition to, children) Dog Moms clearly come from non-Exclusive Dog Mom families. There are Dog Moms in each generation. Is the potential in all of us and only gets switched on in certain individuals? If so, how? Is it a mutation that just keeps popping up at a certain low frequency in the human population regardless of its tendency to lower the fitness of its bearer? I'll be pondering all this in the car on my way to the dog birthday party tomorrow.

Bibliography

Alberto & Troutman. *Applied Behavior Analysis for Teachers 7th Edition* (Prentice Hall, 2005)

Baron-Cohen et al. *Understanding Other Minds: Perspectives from Cognitive Developmental Neuroscience* (Oxford University Press, 2000)

Bekoff, M. "Play Signals as Punctuation: the Structure of Social Play in Canids." *Behaviour*, 132, 419 (1995)

Bekoff & Allen. "Intentional Communication and Social Play: How and Why Animals Negotiate and Agree to Play." In: Bekoff & Byers, eds. *Animal Play* (Cambridge: Cambridge University Press, 1998)

Bolhuis & Giraldeau, eds. *The Behavior of Animals: Mechanism, Function and Evolution* (Wiley, 2004)

Bradley, Janis. *Dogs Bite But Balloons and Slippers Are More Dangerous* (James & Kenneth, 2005)

Call et al. "Domestic Dogs (Canis familiaris) Are Sensitive to the Attentional State of Humans." *Journal of Comparative Psychology*, 117–3, 257–263 (2003)

Carroll, Sean B. *The Making of the Fittest: DNA and the Ultimate Forensic Record of Evolution* (WW Norton, 2007)

Christensen et al. "Aggressive Behavior in Adopted Dogs That Passed a Temperament Test." *Applied Animal Behavior Science*, 106, 85 (2007)

Coppinger & Coppinger. *Dogs: A New Understanding of Canine Origin, Behavior and Evolution* (University of Chicago Press, 2002)

Dawkins, Richard. *The Selfish Gene—30th Anniversary Edition* (Oxford University Press, 2003)

Dawkins, Richard. *Climbing Mount Improbable* (Penguin, 2006)

Dawkins, Richard. *Unweaving the Rainbow* (Penguin, 2006)

Dennett, Daniel. "Intentional Systems in Cognitive Ethology: The Panglossian Paradigm Defended." *The Behavioral and Brain Sciences*, 6, 343 (1983)

Dennett, Daniel. "The Baldwin Effect: A Crane, Not a Skyhook." In: *Evolution and Learning: The Baldwin Effect Reconsidered* (MIT Press, 2002)

Dobney & Larson. "Genetics and Animal Domestication: New Windows on an Elusive Process." *Journal of Zoology*, 269, 261 (2006)

Dunbar, Ian. *How to Teach a New Dog Old Tricks* (James & Kenneth, 1998)

Duxbury et al. "Evaluation of Association Between Retention in the Home and Attendance at Puppy Socialization Classes." *JAVMA*, 223, 1, 61 (2003)

Friedman & Brinker. *The Struggle for Dominance: Fact or Fiction.* Gabrial Foundation website: www.thegabrielfoundation.org.

Hare et al. "The Domestication of Social Cognition in Dogs." *Science*, 298 (2002)

Hauser, Marc D. *Wild Minds: What Animals Really Think* (Henry Holt & Co., 2000)

Kass et al. "Understanding Animal Companion Surplus in the United States: Relinquishment of Nonadoptables to Animal Shelters for Euthanasia." *JAAWS* 4(4), 237 (2001)

Leonard et al. "Ancient DNA Evidence for Old-World Origin of New World Dogs." *Science* 298, 1613 (2002)

Marcus, Gary. *The Birth of the Mind* (Basic Books, 2004)

Mech & Boitani. *Wolves—Behavior, Ecology and Conservation* (University of Chicago Press, 2006)

Meyer & Ladewig. "The Relationship Between Number of Training Sessions per Week and Learning in Dogs." *Applied Animal Behavior Science* (2007)

Meyer & Quenzer. *Psychopharmacology: Drugs, the Brain and Behavior* (Sinauer Associates, 2004)

Miklosi et al. "Use of Experimenter-given Cues in Dogs." *Animal Cognition* 1, 113–122 (1998)

Mills et al, eds. *Current Issues and Research in Veterinary Behavioral Medicine* (Purdue University Press, 2005)

Mineka and Ohman. "Phobias and Preparedness: The Selective, Automatic and Encapsulated Nature of Fear." *Biological Psychiatry*, 52, 927 (2002)

O'Heare, James. *Aggressive Behavior in Dogs—A Comprehensive Technical Manual for Professionals* (Gentle Solutions, 2007)

Ostrander et al, eds. *The Dog and its Genome* (Cold Spring Harbor Laboratory Press, 2006)

Parker et al. "Genetic Structure of the Purebred Domestic Dog." *Science*, 304, 1160 (2004)

Pinker, Steven. *The Stuff of Thought* (Viking Adult, 2007)

Pinker, Steven. *The Blank Slate* (Penguin, 2003)

Pongracz et al. "Preference for Copying Unambiguous Demonstrations in Dogs." *Journal of Comparative Psychology*, 117, 3, 337 (2003)

Pongracz et al. "Social Learning in Dogs: the Effect of a Human Demonstrator on the Performance of Dogs in a Detour Task." *Animal Behavior*, 62, 6 (2001)

Premack & Premack. *Original Intelligence: Unlocking the Mystery of Who We Are* (Boooksurge, 2007)

Premack & Woodruff. "Does the Chimpanzee Have a Theory of Mind?" *Behavioral and Brain Sciences*, 1, 4, 515 (1978)

Pryor, Karen. *Don't Shoot the Dog* (Bantam Books, 2002)

Rescorla, Robert. "Pavlovian Conditioning: It's Not What You Think." *American Psychologist*, 43, 3, 151 (1988)

Ridley, Mark. *Evolution* (Wiley, 2003)

Ridley, Matt. *Genome: Autobiography or a Species in 23 Chapters* (Fourth Estate, 2000)

Ridley, Matt. *Nature Via Nurture* (Harper Perennial, 2004)

Ridley, Matt. *The Origins of Virtue* (Penguin, 1998)

Sagan, Carl. *The Demon-Haunted World: Science as a Candle in the Dark* (Ballantyne Books, 1997)

Salman et al. "Behavioral Reasons for Relinquishment of Dogs and Cats to 12 Shelters." *JAAWS* 3(2), 93 (2000)

Savolainen et al. "Genetic Evidence for an East Asian Origin of Domestic Dogs." *Science*, 298, 1613 (2002)

Savolainen et al. "A Detailed Picture of the Origin of the Australian Dingo, Obtained from the Study of Mitochondrial DNA." *Proceedings of the National Academy of Science*, 101,12387–12390 (2004)

Schalke et al. "Clinical Signs Caused by the Use of Electric Training Collars on Dogs in Everyday Life Situations." *Applied Animal Behavior Science* Special Issue "Veterinary Behavioural Medicine (2006)

Schwarz et al. *Psychology of Learning and Behavior 5th Edition* (WW Norton, 2002)

Serpell, J., ed. *The Domestic Dog: Its Evolution, Behavior and Interactions with People* (Cambridge University Press, 1996)
Shettleworth, Sara. *Cognition, Evolution and Behavior* (Oxford University Press, 1998)

Smith, PK. "Does Play Matter? Functional and Evolutionary Concepts of Animal and Human Play." *The Behavioral and Brain Sciences*, 5, 139 (1992)

Soproni et al. "Dogs' (Canis familiaris) Responsiveness to Human Pointing Gestures." *Journal of Comparative Psychology*, 116-1 (2002)

Svartberg, K. "Breed-typical Behavior in Dogs—Historical Remnants or Recent Constructs?" *Applied Animal Behavior Science*, 96 (2006)

Vas et al. "A Friend or Enemy? Dogs' Reaction to an Unfamiliar Person Showing Behavioural Cues of Threat and Friendliness at Different Times." *Applied Animal Behavior Science*, 94, 99 (2005)

Wright, Robert. *The Moral Animal* (Peter Smith Publisher, 1997)

Zimmer, Carl. *Evolution: The Triumph of an Idea* (Harper Perennial, 2006)

Index

From Dogwise Publishing, www.dogwise.com, 1-800-776-2665

BEHAVIOR & TRAINING

ABC's of Behavior Shaping; Fundamentals of Training; Proactive Behavior Mgmt, DVD. Ted Turner

Aggression In Dogs: Practical Mgmt, Prevention & Behaviour Modification. Brenda Aloff

Am I Safe? DVD. Sarah Kalnajs

Barking. The Sound of a Language. Turid Rugaas

Behavior Problems in Dogs, 3rd ed. William Campbell

Brenda Aloff's Fundamentals: Foundation Training for Every Dog, DVD. Brenda Aloff

Bringing Light to Shadow. A Dog Trainer's Diary. Pam Dennison

Canine Body Language. A Photographic Guide to the Native Language of Dogs. Brenda Aloff

Clicked Retriever. Lana Mitchell

Dog Behavior Problems. The Counselor's Handbook. William Campbell

Dog Detectives. Train Your Dog to Find Lost Pets. Kat Albrecht

Dog Friendly Gardens, Garden Friendly Dogs. Cheryl Smith

Dog Language, An Encyclopedia of Canine Behavior. Roger Abrantes

Evolution of Canine Social Behavior, 2nd ed. Roger Abrantes

Fighting Dominance in a Dog Whispering World, DVD. Jean Donaldson and Ian Dunbar

Focus Not Fear. Training Insights from a Reactive Dog Class. Ali Brown

Give Them a Scalpel and They Will Dissect a Kiss, DVD. Ian Dunbar

Guide To Professional Dog Walking And Home Boarding. Dianne Eibner

Language of Dogs, DVD. Sarah Kalnajs

Mastering Variable Surface Tracking, Component Tracking (2 bk set). Ed Presnall

Mindful Dog Teaching: Reflections on the Relationships We Share with our Dogs. Claudeen McAuliffe

My Dog Pulls. What Do I Do? Turid Rugaas

New Knowledge of Dog Behavior (reprint). Clarence Pfaffenberger

On Talking Terms with Dogs: Calming Signals, 2nd edition. Turid Rugaas

On Talking Terms with Dogs: What Your Dog Tells You, DVD. Turid Rugaas

Positive Perspectives: Love Your Dog, Train Your Dog. Pat Miller

Positive Perspectives 2: Know Your Dog, Train Your Dog. Pat Miller

Positive Training for Show Dogs: Building a Relationship for Success. Vicki Ronchette

Predation and Family Dogs, DVD. Jean Donaldson

Really Reliable Recall. Train Your Dog to Come When Called, DVD. Leslie Nelson

Right on Target. Taking Dog Training to a New Level. Mandy Book & Cheryl Smith

Stress in Dogs. Martina Scholz & Clarissa von Reinhardt

The Dog Trainer's Resource: The APDT Chronicle of the Dog Collection. Mychelle Blake (*ed*)

Therapy Dogs: Training Your Dog To Reach Others. Kathy Diamond Davis

Training Dogs, A Manual (reprint). Konrad Most

Training the Disaster Search Dog. Shirley Hammond

Try Tracking: The Puppy Tracking Primer. Carolyn Krause

Visiting the Dog Park, Having Fun, and Staying Safe. Cheryl S. Smith

When Pigs Fly. Train Your Impossible Dog. Jane Killion

Winning Team. A Guidebook for Junior Showmanship. Gail Haynes

Working Dogs (reprint). Elliot Humphrey & Lucien Warner

HEALTH & ANATOMY, SHOWING

An Eye for a Dog. Illustrated Guide to Judging Purebred Dogs. Robert Cole

Annie On Dogs! Ann Rogers Clark

Canine Cineradiography, DVD. Rachel Page Elliott

Canine Massage: A Complete Reference Manual. Jean-Pierre Hourdebaigt

Canine Terminology (reprint). Harold Spira

Dog In Action (reprint). Macdowell Lyon

Dogsteps DVD. Rachel Page Elliott

Performance Dog Nutrition: Optimize Performance With Nutrition. Jocelynn Jacobs

Puppy Intensive Care: A Breeder's Guide To Care Of Newborn Puppies. Myra Savant Harris

Raw Dog Food: Make It Easy for You and Your Dog. Carina MacDonald

Raw Meaty Bones. Tom Lonsdale

Shock to the System. The Facts About Animal Vaccination... Catherine O'Driscoll

The History and Management of the Mastiff. Elizabeth Baxter & Pat Hoffman

Work Wonders. Feed Your Dog Raw Meaty Bones. Tom Lonsdale

Whelping Healthy Puppies, DVD. Sylvia Smart